"Most of the literature on sexual boundary violations focuses on the individual psychology of the analyst and the patient. This groundbreaking volume treats the continuing prevalence of boundary violations as a property of the group, focusing steadily on the analyst's transgression as an inherent by-product of the profession itself. What is it about psychoanalysis that breeds ethical misconduct in the name of healing? Is there a cure? This book is riveting, both for its original and well-written scholarship and its direct confrontation of the psychoanalytic field."

Dawn Skorczewski, Ph.D., Research Professor of English, Brandeis University

W0113876

Social Aspects of Sexual Boundary Trouble in Psychoanalysis

Inspired by the clinical and ethical contributions of Muriel Dimen, *Social Aspects of Sexual Boundary Trouble* goes beyond the established consensus that sexual boundary violations (SBV) constitute a serious breach of professional ethics, in order to explore the cultural and historical implications of their chronic persistence.

In *Rotten Apples and Ambivalence*, her last major publication, Dimen (2016) maintained that "the phenomenon of sexual transgression between analyst and patient … is insufficiently addressed so long as it is only deemed psychological." In responding to and developing Dimen's argument, the distinguished contributors to this volume bring the discussion of SBV to a new level of ethical rigor and depth, challenging the psychoanalytic profession to go beyond its codified complacency. This collection shatters normative professional guidelines by focusing on the complicity and hypocrisy of professional groups, while at the same time raising the taboo subject of the ordinary practicing clinician's unconscious professional ambivalence and potentially "rogue" sexual subjectivity.

Social Aspects of Sexual Boundary Trouble uncovers the roots of SBV in the institutional origins and history of psychoanalysis as a profession. Exploring Dimen's concept of the psychoanalytic "primal crime," which is in some ways constitutive of the profession, and the inherently unstable nature of interpersonal and professional "boundaries," *Social Aspects of Sexual Boundary Trouble* breaks new ground in the continuing struggle of psychoanalysis to reconcile itself with its liminal social status and its origins as a subversive, morally ambiguous practice.

It will be highly relevant to specialists in psychoanalysis, psychotherapy, critical theory, feminist studies and social thought.

Charles Levin, Ph.D., F.I.P.A. is a Training and Supervising Analyst, Editor-in-chief, *Canadian Journal of Psychoanalysis*, and Director, Canadian Institute of Psychoanalysis. He has edited and authored several analytic books and many articles on clinical, ethical and cultural topics.

Relational Perspectives Book Series

Adrienne Harris, Steven Kuchuck & Eyal Rozmarin
Series Editors

Stephen Mitchell
Founding Editor

Lewis Aron
Editor Emeritus

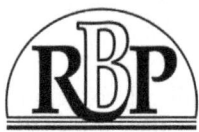

The Relational Perspectives Book Series (RPBS) publishes books that grow out of or contribute to the relational tradition in contemporary psychoanalysis. The term *relational psychoanalysis* was first used by Greenberg and Mitchell[1] to bridge the traditions of interpersonal relations, as developed within interpersonal psychoanalysis and object relations, as developed within contemporary British theory. But, under the seminal work of the late Stephen A. Mitchell, the term *relational psychoanalysis* grew and began to accrue to itself many other influences and developments. Various tributaries—interpersonal psychoanalysis, object relations theory, self psychology, empirical infancy research, feminism, queer theory, sociocultural studies and elements of contemporary Freudian and Kleinian thought—flow into this tradition, which understands relational configurations between self and others, both real and fantasied, as the primary subject of psychoanalytic investigation.

We refer to the relational tradition, rather than to a relational school, to highlight that we are identifying a trend, a tendency within contemporary psychoanalysis, not a more formally organized or coherent school or system of beliefs. Our use of the term *relational* signifies a dimension of theory and practice that has become salient across the wide spectrum of contemporary psychoanalysis. Now under the editorial supervision of Adrienne Harris, Steven Kuchuck and Eyal Rozmarin, the Relational Perspectives Book Series originated in 1990 under the editorial eye of the late Stephen A. Mitchell. Mitchell was the most prolific and influential of the originators of the relational tradition. Committed to dialogue among psychoanalysts, he abhorred the authoritarianism that dictated adherence to a rigid set of beliefs or technical restrictions. He championed open discussion, comparative and integrative approaches, and promoted new voices across the generations. Mitchell was later joined by the late Lewis Aron, also a visionary and influential writer, teacher and leading thinker in relational psychoanalysis.

Included in the Relational Perspectives Book Series are authors and works that come from within the relational tradition, those that extend and develop that tradition, and works that critique relational approaches or compare and contrast them with alternative points of view. The series includes our most distinguished senior psychoanalysts, along with younger contributors who bring fresh vision. Our aim is to enable a deepening of relational thinking while reaching across disciplinary and social boundaries in order to foster an inclusive and international literature.

A full list of titles in this series is available at https://www.routledge.com/mentalhealth/series/LEARPBS.

Note

1 Greenberg, J. & Mitchell, S. (1983). *Object relations in psychoanalytic theory.* Cambridge, MA: Harvard University Press.

Social Aspects of Sexual Boundary Trouble in Psychoanalysis

Responses to the Work of Muriel Dimen

Edited by Charles Levin

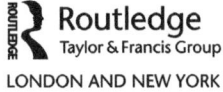

Routledge
Taylor & Francis Group

LONDON AND NEW YORK

First published 2021
by Routledge
2 Park Square, Milton Park, Abingdon, Oxon OX14 4RN

and by Routledge
52 Vanderbilt Avenue, New York, NY 10017

Routledge is an imprint of the Taylor & Francis Group, an informa business

British Library Cataloguing-in-Publication Data
A catalogue record for this book is available from the British Library

Library of Congress Cataloging-in-Publication Data
Names: Levin, Charles, 1950- editor.
Title: Social aspects of sexual boundary trouble in psychoanalysis : responses to the work of Muriel Dimen / edited by Charles Levin.
Description: Abingdon, Oxon ; New York, NY : Routledge, 2021. | Series: Relational perspectives book series | Includes bibliographical references and index. |
Identifiers: LCCN 2020021051 (print) | LCCN 2020021052 (ebook) | ISBN 9780367483784 (hardback) | ISBN 9780367483760 (paperback) | ISBN 9781003039587 (ebook)
Subjects: LCSH: Sex between psychotherapist and patient. | Psychotherapist and patient. | Psychotherapists–Professional ethics. | Psychoanalysis–Moral and ethical aspects. | Dimen, Muriel.
Classification: LCC RC489.S47 S63 2021 (print) | LCC RC489.S47 (ebook) | DDC 616.89/14–dc23
LC record available at https://lccn.loc.gov/2020021051
LC ebook record available at https://lccn.loc.gov/2020021052

ISBN: 978-0-367-48378-4 (hbk)
ISBN: 978-0-367-48376-0 (pbk)
ISBN: 978-1-003-03958-7 (ebk)

Typeset in Times
by River Editorial Ltd, Devon, UK

In memoriam: Muriel Dimen (1942–2016)

Contents

Contributors

Steven Cooper, Ph.D., is Associate Professor of Psychology, Harvard Medical School; Training and Supervising Analyst, the Boston Psychoanalytic Society and Institute; and Joint Chief Editor Emeritus, *Psychoanalytic Dialogues*. His most recent book is *The analyst's experience of the depressive position: The melancholic errand of psychoanalysis* (Routledge).

Terry Davis, Ph.D., is a faculty member of a psychoanalytic institute affiliated with the International Psychoanalytic Association

Muriel Dimen, Ph.D. (1942–2016), was a pioneer in the feminist transformation of the psychoanalytic landscape. Originally trained as an anthropologist, she undertook her personal analysis early in her adult life and continued on to become a major clinical contributor to the rise of relational psychoanalysis in New York. She retired as professor emeritus of anthropology at CUNY and became Adjunct Professor of Clinical Psychology at New York University, teaching and supervising regularly in the Post Doctoral Program in Psychotherapy and Psychoanalysis. She was an Associate Editor of *Psychoanalytic Dialogues*, principal editor of *Studies in Gender and Sexuality*, and founding board member of the International Association for Relational Psychoanalysis and Psychotherapy (IARPP).

Katie Gentile, Ph.D., is Professor of Gender Studies in the Department of Interdisciplinary Studies at John Jay College of Criminal Justice (City University of New York). She is the author of *Creating bodies: Eating disorders as self-destructive survival* and *The*

Business of being made: The temporalities of reproductive technologies in psychoanalysis and cultures, both from Routledge. She the editor of the Routledge book series *Genders & Sexualities in Mind & Culture* and a co-editor of the journal *Studies in Gender and Sexuality.* She is on the faculty of New York University's Post-doctoral Program in Psychotherapy and Psychoanalysis and in private practice in New York City.

Adrienne Harris, Ph.D., is Faculty and Supervisor at New York University Postdoctoral Program in Psychotherapy and Psychoanalysis. She is on the faculty and is a supervisor at the Psychoanalytic Institute of Northern California. She is an Editor at *Psychoanalytic Dialogues,* and *Studies In Gender and Sexuality.* In 2009, She, Lewis Aron, and Jeremy Safran established the Sandor Ferenczi Center at the New School University. With Lew Aron, Eyal Rozmarin and Steven Kuchuck, she co-edits the Book Series *Relational Perspectives in Psychoanalysis,* a series with over 90 published volumes. She is an editor of the IPA ejournal *Psychoanalysistoday.com,* which is developing cross cultural communications on the topics of Violence and Migration. She has written on topics in gender and development, analytic subjectivity and self-care, primitive states and the analytic community in the shadow of the First World War. Her current work is on analytic subjectivity, on intersectional models of gender and sexuality, and on ghosts.

Stephen Hartman, Ph.D., teaches at the Psychoanalytic Institute of Northern California and is a faculty member of the relational track at the NYU Postdoctoral Program in Psychotherapy and Psychoanalysis. He is co-editor of *Studies in Gender and Sexuality,* an associate editor for *Psychoanalytic Dialogues* and a co-editor of the Psychoanalytic Dialogues Blog.

Charles Levin, Ph.D., FIPA, is Director of the Canadian Institute of Psychoanalysis (C.I.P.) and Director of the CIP-affiliated English psychoanalytic training program in Montreal. He is Editor-in-chief, *Canadian Journal of Psychoanalysis/Revue canadienne de psychanalyse,* and author, editor and collaborator on many psychoanalytic books and articles addressing clinical, ethical and cultural topics, including *Confidentiality: Ethical perspectives and clinical dilemmas*

(Analytic Press, 2003) and *Art in the offertorium: Narcissism, psychoanalysis and cultural metaphysics* (Rodopi 2012).

Ann Pellegrini, Ph.D., is Professor of Performance Studies and Social and Cultural Analysis at New York University. Her books include *Performance Anxieties: Staging Psychoanalysis, Staging Race* (Routledge, 1997); *Love the Sin: Sexual Regulation and the Limits of Religious Tolerance* (New York University Press, 2003), co-authored with Janet R. Jakobsen; *Secularisms* (Duke University Press, 2008), co-edited with Jakobsen; and *"You Can Tell Just By Looking" and 21 Other Myths About LGBT Life and People* (Beacon, 2013), co-authored with Michael Bronski and Michael Amico. She is co-editor of the "Sexual Cultures" book series at New York University Press, and a contributing editor to the journal *Studies in Gender and Sexuality.*

Avgi Saketopoulou, Ph.D., is faculty at NYU Postdoctoral Program in Psychotherapy and Psychoanalysis, the William Allanson White Institute, the New York Psychoanalytic Institute, the National Institute for the Psychotherapies, the Stephen Mitchell Relational Center and the Chicago Center for Psychoanalysis. She serves on the editorial boards of the *Journal of the American Psychoanalytic Association (JAPA), Psychoanalytic Dialogues* and *Studies in Gender and Sexuality (SGS)*. She has received several awards, including the Ruth Stein prize, the Roughton award from the American Psychoanalytic Association, the Symonds prize from SGS and the JAPA annual prize. Dr. Saketopoulou has published work on trauma and its representation, on traumatic and normative gender, on psychosexuality and perversion and on the enigmatics of consent.

Acknowledgments

Muriel Dimen and her work were the inspiration for this book, which is dedicated to her memory. I will always cherish the friendship we had. I am also very grateful to my collaborators, the contributors to this book, many of whom were close to Muriel. They have been brilliant, generous, diligent and kind.

This collection of essays came together through much dialogue among the participants, and a great deal of personal struggle on their part, in response to some of the most difficult clinical and ethical issues facing our profession. In the end, it proved impossible to contain their number and enthusiasm in one volume of tribute to Muriel's work, and so the project had to be split in two, causing some unexpected delay. The present collection, *Social Aspects of Sexual Boundary Violations in Psychoanalysis: Responses to the Work of Muriel Dimen,* emphasizes the systemic nature of the ethical problems in psychoanalytic groups and communities. Its companion, *Sexual Boundary Trouble in Psychoanalysis: Clinical Perspectives on Muriel Dimen's Concept of the "Primal Crime,"* emphasizes the clinical implications of her work. Each of the chapters in both collections grew from a remarkable sense of purpose and mission, of which I was the privileged witness and beneficiary. In particular I want to thank Adrienne Harris, whose sympathy, patience, encouragement, and dedication have been essential to me in the preparation of both volumes. I am also very grateful to the Executors of Muriel Dimen's literary estate, Virginia Goldner and Avgi Saketopoulou, for their gracious assistance and guidance in the editing process, and for their permission to use Muriel's last published paper in this collection.

The idea that it would be a good thing for the analytic community, which includes our patients, to publish a discussion inspired by Muriel Dimen's (2011) account of her own analysis, *Lapsus Linguae*, owes much to IARPP, and also to Mark Blechner. At that time he was the editor of *Contemporary Psychoanalysis,* and willing to publish Muriel's seminal text, when other editors found it too long and controversial. This was perhaps the first time that a psychoanalyst had dared, in a non-sensational way, to discuss the less savory details of her own analysis in public.

In 2011, the International Association of Relational Psychoanalysts and Psychotherapists (IARPP) held an internet Colloquium on the topic of Muriel Dimen's paper, *Lapsus Linguae.* Katie Gentile and Eyal Rozmarin were the brilliant moderators of that powerful and contentious, sometimes stormy Colloquium. All of the people involved in that IARPP project deserve a great deal of credit. Not least among them are the many analytic patients who contributed important and illuminating personal accounts of their analytic experiences. Many of them, like Muriel, were also analysts. The whole IARPP community, as gathered for that occasion, did something very special and unusual that prompted me to imagine this book.

I am not the only author and editor in our field who is indebted to Kate Hawes and her remarkable team at Routledge. Kate is a bit of an enigma to me. How can she be so patient, and so forgiving? What I have learned is that she is personally very dedicated to keeping psychoanalysis happening. Kate's staff at Taylor and Francis, especially Hannah Wright, whose editorial stewardship has been impeccable, reflect this embracing spirit. I also want to mention the editors of the Relational Perspectives Series, Adrienne Harris, Steven Kuchuk, Eyal Rozmarin, and the late, great Lew Aron.

The editors of *Psychoanalytic Dialogues,* and *The American Journal of Psychoanalysis* were very generous in granting permission to republish the material appearing in the following chapters:

Chapter 2 was originally published in *Journal of the American Psychoanalytic Association* 64(2): 361–373 (2016).

Portions of Chapter 4 appeared previously in Harris, A. and Gentile, K. (2019). Boundary violations, consent, the law, and the lawless, in P. Montagna and A. Harris (Eds.), *Psychoanalysis, Law, and Society* (pp. 108–122). London and New York: Routledge. They are reprinted here with permission.

Parts of Chapter 7 appeared previously in Steven Cooper, *The Analyst's Experience of the Depressive Position,* New York & London: Routledge, 2016; and in *Psychoanalytic Dialogues* 26(2): 206–214 (2016). They are reprinted here with permission.

One more thing: thank you, my darling Kathi.

Chapter 1

Introduction

Social preconditions of psycho-sexual violations in psychoanalysis: reflections on the ethics of Muriel Dimen

Charles Levin

Psychoanalysts are people who by definition believe it important to be willing and able to examine themselves and to take responsibility for the way they live their lives. We even believe that we should, like our analysands, be open to letting others help us in the process of self-exploration. Psychoanalysis is a social relationship—if an odd and enigmatic one.

At the same time, analysts believe in "freedom" and "independence": personal autonomy in the sense that we all strive for moral integrity, which requires expressive freedom, privacy, and clear definitions of our ethical responsibilities. Analysts are especially trained to recognize the individual damage created by mental enslavement to intrusive, controlling, or neglectful dependency figures (internal objects), especially in formative periods of life. We want our patients to be able to think for themselves and we personally aspire to the same ideal.

But one fact of our institutional life seems to throw these comfortable, albeit demanding assumptions askew: the persistence of sexual boundary violations (SBV). Boundary violations force us to tangle in a personal way with something that exceeds the grasp of psychoanalytic "training" as it currently exists.

Boundary violations cause serious moral harm within the entire psychoanalytic community, even when they go undetected. The community that is affected includes not only analysts; it is also made up of patients, their families, friends, their *pith* and their *kith* (Ross, 1995). Psychoanalysis involves a wider and deeper social network than we may prefer at times to imagine, whose boundaries are indeterminate.

So the fact of SBV requires us to expand our sense of community. In this vertex, the occurrence of SBV offers itself as an interpretation of group behavior. We are not likely to receive this interpretation gladly, of course; we may want to get rid of it in some way, because it threatens to undermine our sense of who we are, what we are, and who or what is "them." The persistence of boundary violations confronts the members of the psychoanalytic profession with a moral demand—a responsibility—that perhaps few of us believe we freely chose. When becoming an analyst, we don't usually say to ourselves, "I want to (or I will) be responsible for the malpractice committed by other analysts." It would seem to us absurd to be morally saddled in that way. However, even before our profession became especially concerned about sexual misconduct (which was often tolerated and covered up by institutes), we have always tacitly agreed to a form of collective responsibility in the sense that we should, of course, regulate ourselves and even police ourselves. (For a cogent critique of this concept of self-policing, see Gentile, this volume.) Initially, institutionalized psychoanalysis believed (along the lines of Plato's *Republic* [see Levin, this volume]) that we could accomplish this goal simply by choosing the right people to become analysts, making sure that they get properly analysed (hence the hierarchical training analyst system), imposing burdensome requirements, and establishing rigorous and even rigid rules for psychoanalytic education ("training").

Round about the mid-1980s, however (in what I call the "Gabbard Revolution"), we began to realize that psychoanalysis had an image problem and that we needed, at the very least, to demonstrate, in public, that justice was being done. This was the beginning of a long slippery slope in which we have conceded more and more of our sovereignty to the demands of the other. In that era, we drew up and published codes of ethics and created channels for complaint-driven ethical review of our colleagues. We began to think about our own behavior in terms of psychoanalytic principles (a novel idea), challenging morally lackadaisical attitudes and self-serving rationalizations, to the point where it actually became, for example, much more difficult to marry a patient (hitherto a common practice) while retaining peer respect. Above all, we made a show of punishing "offenders," frequently by banishing them. But the problem still didn't go away, as Glen Gabbard (2017) lamented, after thirty years of research and consulting on the issue, in a searing and pessimistic review of the problem. Gabbard found no evidence that anything we have done about the problem so far has contributed to the prevention of SBV. This suggests that Muriel Dimen put her finger on something very important when she wrote, in a revealing phrase, that "psychoanalytic life is burdened by a routine dissociation" (2016, p. 370; this volume, p. 39).

Part I: collective responsibility for the primal crime

The essays in this collection start from Muriel Dimen's premise that psychoanalytic responsibility for boundary violations is not only moral in nature, it is also social. As Gabbard and numerous others originally recognized, psychoanalysis not only has a public interface; it is itself a kind of social system embedded within the larger society—a social system that we have been reluctant, over several generations of analytic practice, to carefully examine. Not only are boundary violations a part of that social system; the way we handle or mishandle them as a group is symptomatic of that system.

All of Dimen's arguments about SBV assume our collective moral responsibility—not just *when* SBVs occur, but *for their occurrence in general*. Something needs to be done *by the group* beyond the deliberative exercise of determining whether a violation has occurred and meting out justice. What many consider special about Dimen's work is that she pushes the implications of the idea of collective responsibility to the point where we find ourselves in unknown territory, somewhere beyond the conceptual site of the Gabbard Revolution. How to explain this?

Reflecting on Dimen's psychoanalytic work, I think we can see now more clearly how she first shifted the argument and raised it up a notch, particularly through the vertex of feminism and social anthropology, her concomitant areas of expertise. Dimen (2011) showed that our collective responsibility for boundary violations includes an element of collusion, what might be described as tacit participation in a social dynamic of denial and dissociation. The dynamic in question is really a vicious circle in which the group turns a (half-) blind eye to the problem and thus, in various ways, feeds back into it. That dynamic functions on several levels involving the systemic inequalities and biases characteristic of modern patriarchy. Though partially mitigated by law in complex liberal democracies, patriarchy is widely ramified in specialized systems and reproduces itself easily. The psychoanalytic profession is one of these systems.

As members of the psychoanalytic group, we have expected that our professional education, combined with stiff sanctions for ethical infractions, would have a deterrent effect on SBV. Yet the manner in which we address the problem—secretive, defensive, formalistic, administrative—does not inspire hope. There is a general sense of alienation in the profession, and the continuing reluctance or inability of the group and its leaders to deal with serious violations openly increases the sense of distrust and generates a pervasive feeling of inauthenticity. The leaders themselves are often prey to the alienation and even become public role models of cynicism. Indeed, the annals of psychoanalytic atrocity are heavily weighted with its more distinguished members. For these reasons, the seeming inauthenticity of ethics investigations into SBV may actually transfigure the crime into an unconsciously preferred vehicle for other members who are struggling with the impulse to rebel. We all have such motives! The table is then set for the next round of scandal; all that is required to complete another cycle is the statistically inevitable personal crisis that will crop up somewhere within the membership body.

It is in this perspective that Dimen defines SBV as a property of the psychoanalytic group (2016, p. 362; this volume, p. 29 passim). All of her work, even when not devoted specifically to psychoanalytic ethics, suggests that seemingly individual problems—for example, certain kinds of negative ("counter")-transference that regulate conventional boundaries between normal and pathological, or healthy and perverse—cannot be addressed responsibly when the underlying social structure and dynamic are kept out of view (Dimen, 2003, 2005).

An occupational hazard of psychoanalysis is to see everything in psychological terms. In *Rotten Apples and Ambivalence*, Dimen comments: "the phenomenon of sexual transgression between analyst and patient … is insufficiently addressed so long as it is only deemed psychological" (2016, p. 361; this volume, p. 29). Dimen made systematically explicit in this paper what she had previously explored in her earlier, partly autobiographical reflections (2011; see also Levin, 2020a), namely, that the phenomena of sexual transgression in psychoanalysis are "also workings of power and vehicles of culture." To address them adequately, she argued, one needs to "think socially," and to provide not only an "insider" account of the problem (as she had done before, writing as an analyst and as a patient victim of SBV), but also to take a multi-perspectival look "from the outside in" (2016, p. 361; this volume, p. 29).

This line of thinking suggests a number of troubling questions about how we (the profession) have handled the issue so far. In effect, Dimen is asking, was it even true that we took our moral, if not quite our social, responsibility seriously? One reason for this question, she clearly implies, but did not live long enough to fully articulate, is that even in the *thought* of our collective responsibility, we have tailored our ethics along individualistic, one-person psychology lines that do not in any profound way challenge the basic feeling of non-involvement that we manage to sustain even as we assume this new (and hopefully developing) sense of collective responsibility.

We know from the histories of North and South America, and of modern colonialism generally, which spanned the globe, including Africa, Asia, the "Middle" East, and Europe itself, that nations and cultures have been built on foundations of generalized violence. Muriel Dimen's (2014) reflections on the early institutionalization of psychoanalysis suggest that we can learn a great deal by looking at the development of our profession through a similar historical lens. As Dimen noted, Freud's announcement of the inception of the IPA, with the justifications he provided for it, simultaneously "declares a revolution and forges an orthodoxy" (Dimen, 2014, p. 499). The idea that psychoanalytic institutions were established by means of a kind of violent schismogenesis[1] lies at the root of what she was getting at, I believe, in her important, but neglected concept of the psychoanalytic "primal crime" (Dimen, 2011; see Levin, 2020a, 2020b). The fact that many typical creation myths involve narratives of violent splitting (e.g. the *tzintzum* in the Lurianic *Kabbalah*, or the story in *Genesis* about Adam's rib) does not derogate from the ethical need for the parties so engendered, in the real world, to keep in mind the likelihood of originary violence at the root of their sense of "identity." And why wouldn't we? The answer may be that Freud's assertion on our behalf of psychoanalysis as a "new movement" (1914, p. 42) whose achievement must be enshrined by orthodoxy in the IPA "headquarters" (1914, p. 43), conceals yet another, still more "primal" violence that we do not wish to remember: the socially transgressive undertones of the psychoanalytic procedure itself—the fact that in spite of Freud's later protestations to the contrary (Freud, 1910), psychoanalysis is inherently "wild."

As Freud (1912) inferred from the hypothesis of the "primal horde" in his philosophical reconstruction of human cultural origins (*Totem and Taboo*), there must have been a critical moment after which "society was now based on complicity in the common crime" (p. 146). Modern cultural anthropology has rightly questioned the validity of Freud's speculations about human pre-history, but he nonetheless significantly shifted our intellectual ground by suggesting that, whatever the status of violence in the human picture we draw, our authoritarian tendencies can be understood as defensive as opposed to essential or innate. We also learn from Freud that what is most significant over the long term about the moral fact of violence in the process of "nation building" is that the constitutive violence is not only forgotten, its memory suppressed; but also that the violence itself is defensively folded into the culture and ongoing practice of the "nation" as a whole, and the world: it has no other place to go. Originary violence is lived unconsciously and/or vicariously through attitudes, customs, norms and ideals that are taken at face value, though they refract and institutionalize, in subtle ways, the suppressed history.

Not all of what is refracted in the roots of our various collective identities—professional, cultural, ethnic, racial—takes the form of overt social actions in the sense we traditionally define as history and politics. There are areas of human activity that escape our conscious notice. We might describe them more broadly as trans-individual rather than "social" or "societal" in the conventional sense. These liminal and/or unconscious activities have only recently begun to draw the interest of human self-research (psychology, sociology, anthropology, history, evolutionary thought). Try as we might, they resist location on the grids of internal versus external or individual versus social; and they are deeply implicated in our origins and the sense of who we are as psychoanalysts.

Freud not only understood this, he contributed mightily to the development of such a perspective in human cultural evolution, which arguably adds more than his ideas about clinical treatment to the weight of psychoanalysis in our intellectual universe. The implicit analogy of Freud (1912, 1939) recognized that in some way (not necessarily precisely in the forms he speculated), human cultures in general are grounded in sexuality and violence, in the problematics of incest and the dynamics of murder within the group.[2] This supra-individual and proto-social aspect of sexuality and violence sets Freud's anthropological speculations apart from earlier theories about the social contract and the state of nature. For Freud, at least by implication, the ways that humans have come to socially organize sexuality and violence are not merely naturalized events belonging to an evolutionary past or a biological heritage—they are ongoing elements of cultural evolution in history as it unfolds in our present lives.

To proceed somewhat programmatically, in the interests of space: the sense of our social responsibility for sexual boundary violations has been suppressed within psychoanalysis at a number of levels. In summary, these include at least three interrelated forms of foundational schismogenesis: 1) the founding of psychoanalytic institutions on the basis of patriarchal and authoritarian models of governance and education dating back to Plato's *Republic*, which inhibit freedom of thought; 2) the forging of a professional identity with respect to medicine, psychology, and conventional social thought through forms of group consolidation and control—the "submissive transformation of narcissism" (Levin, 2021b)—harkening back to the Exodus myth and Moses' divine mission to lead the "chosen" people; 3) asserting the concept of unconscious sexuality as a specific "object domain" proper to psychoanalysis alone and its specialized technique; but then absolving itself from the implications of that understanding of sexuality (see Saketopoulou, this volume)—first, by claiming professional immunity from it (through specialized theory and technique); and then by subsuming sexuality itself into a larger paradigm of individual emotional development (psychosexual stages, object relations, attachment theory, etc.).

To develop these points a bit further, we might say that Dimen's work tends toward a redefinition of the concept of sexual boundary violation, a revisioning in which the ambiguous and indeterminate role of sexuality is recognized. As we have already considered, Dimen's concept of the "primal crime" invites us to revisit the status of sexual boundaries at the historical beginnings of psychoanalysis. What is a sexual boundary, after all? We know that the required intimacy of the analytic relationship was widely considered improper in the early days of psychoanalysis, "a most dangerous method," as William James opined (on this topic, see especially Kerr [1993]). Consideration of the porousness of the frame at that time suggests to us now that psychic "boundaries" should really be thought of as both psychosexual and sociocultural constructs. In the early days of psychoanalysis, as we know, confidentiality about patients was not maintained between colleagues (e.g., Freud reported to Jones frequently on his analysis of Jones' mistress, Loe Kann) and the incest taboo was widely flouted (e.g., Freud analysed his own daughter, Klein analysed her children). (On Freud and Klein analysing their own offspring, see respectively Young-Bruehl [1988] and Grosskurth [1998]. On Jonesian sexual misbehavior, see Maddox [2006]). In the late 1890s, Freud's emerging conceptualization of psychoanalysis and of the place of sexuality in the genesis of psychic life had led him further and further onto the other side of a social boundary that was both personal and sexual. The conclusion is inescapable that psychoanalysis itself could not have come into existence other than as a psychosexual violation of social boundaries; and in that sense, "boundary violation" as a term refers to a dynamic that is constitutive of psychoanalysis (see also Hartman, this volume).

From this perspective, speaking to the first two of the three problematics listed above, the breach of psychosexual boundaries no longer appears as an aberration from the psychoanalytic norm, but as an important aspect of its founding moment (crudely put, in Freud's ingenious repurposing of patriarchal control over the "hysterical" female body). Likewise, the breaching of boundaries emerges as a defining feature of collective psychoanalytic identity. Not only does Freud, like Moses, lead his followers out of the darkness toward the promised land of sexual enlightenment; he imposes a rigid hierarchal "rule of law" over the teaching and practice of psychoanalysis (see Levin, this volume). Finally, through Dimen's perspective, the third problematic comes into view, namely that psychoanalysis became "a host to crucial tensions" (Dimen, 2014, p. 499): perpetually at odds with itself, caught between "civilization and its discontents," psychoanalysis becomes a kind of "acivilization" (Levin, 2000), parrying its own essential truths in an impossible project of self-legitimation, in which it simultaneously asserts and denies the primacy of sexuality in its theory, its practice, and its institutional organization.

In the traditional picture of SBV, sexuality figures as a powerful independent force. If the analyst is personally vulnerable (or psychopathic, or poorly trained and analysed), he or she is at great risk of enacting ethically inappropriate sexual scenarios with the patient. In this model, the individual patient is the victim, the individual analyst is the perpetrator, and the psychoanalytic profession is only responsible in a limited sense—it must decide on the professional fate of its member. Dimen (2016, this volume) characterizes this model as the "rotten apple" theory. If we throw out the bad apple and everybody takes a shower, we all come out feeling relatively clean, if a little shaken.

Dimen's alternative picture of SBV suggests a range of important issues and responsibilities that are largely ignored in the rotten apple perspective. There is of course the thorny question of the profession's responsibilities to the patient-victim. In the rotten apple perspective, the obligation to make some kind of reparation to the victim, if any, usually falls on the shoulders of the designated transgressor alone. Justice is achieved in retributive rather than restorative or reparative action, and the analytic group is not called upon to account for itself in any definite way (apart from publically condemning the breach of ethics). The opportunity for the group to learn something (possibly valuable) from its former member (who in many cases is a training analyst and a revered teacher, leader, supervisor, and author)—and also from the victim—is usually sabotaged by the threat of legal liability attached to any form of open or spontaneous communication between the parties (victim, transgressor, group). Yet one wonders in many cases if these legal obstacles might have been overcome if there were not already a powerful self-serving incentive on the part of the profession to avoid the risk of recognizing itself in what happened between the transgressor and the victim. The occurrence of SBV tends to split the analytic group into warring political factions allergic to self-reflection.

With overt transgression, social bonds that had once existed between the parties (patient, analyst, group) are severed, or severely damaged. There is ostracization or excommunication, often exacerbated by the defensive withdrawal of the accused analyst, who hides in shame behind a veil of legal self-interest and prevarication. But the analytic group does the same thing. Legal advice, considerations of confidentiality, the threat of lawsuits all serve as a cover for what is arguably an evasion of ethical responsibility on the part of the group (see, for example, Sundelson, 2003). Both sides want to distance themselves as quickly and cleanly as possible from the victim. Neither side wants to look the other in the eye. Neither side wants to face any awkward questions: How did this happen? Why did it happen? Who are you? Who am I? *What* are we?

To reframe this problem somewhat, we might imagine a generic situation, a kind of collective fantasy (one which I would argue reflects the origins of psychoanalysis in perceived or imagined violence):

A patient has a complaint about psychoanalysis.

This proposition bespeaks an underground situation of long standing—one characterised by the broad form of the "routine dissociation" that Dimen (2016) describes. On the professional side, routine dissociation is surely rooted in every psychoanalyst's unconscious alarm at the very idea of getting inside another mind, and the possibilities such getting would afford. In historical fact, the fear that psychoanalysis must face a complaint made against it is as old as the analytic literature itself, dating back to the stories of Anna O and Dora (Breuer & Freud, 1893–1895; Freud, 1905).

Schematically, in the standard variant of this narrative, the patient has a complaint about psychoanalysis and does not know where to go with it. The analyst reveals to the patient that it is precisely to the analyst the patient must come with the complaint—that the complaint is in effect a statement of the problem the patient needs to work out. All kinds of different scenarios may follow on from this. The patient may have felt that the only way to get the attention of the analyst was to formulate their complaint in sexual terms, often as a demand for love. The analyst may then be able to work with the complaint in a way that helps the patient to feel heard and to resolve the complaint. This is the traditional transference model. But, as we know, it has another common variation: the patient has a complaint about psychoanalysis but it is the analyst who implicitly or explicitly reformulates the complaint in terms of the patient's sexual desire for the analyst, perhaps in order to concentrate the attention of the patient or to regain the high ground. The patient responds in these terms, but then may feel misunderstood, or devalued and rejected. Whatever the case, things are liable to get out of hand, at which point some sort of sexual encounter may very well ensue. In many but not all cases, the patient later regrets the loss and betrayal of the analytic relationship, and redirects the complaint to the community at large in terms of a sexual boundary violation.

There are many intervening plotlines in this psychoanalytic day-dream, oscillating between psychoanalytic vindication and professional ignominy. The permutations of the storyline are reminiscent of Freud's (1919) structural analysis of beating fantasies (including those of his daughter Anna)—the versions that can be remembered and those that remain unconscious. One can imagine how anxious and defensive the early analysts must have felt, armed with a theory of unconscious sexuality, and attempting to practice this new experimental human relationship on live subjects. How would they tolerate the risks? And what would become of them if anything went wrong? They had only Freud's say so to go on, which is surely a reason why loyalty to him was so important in the early days. But Freud was himself dealing with these risks in a counter-phobic way, as if to convince himself that the technique was completely neutral (I could even analyse my own child). If one thinks along the generic lines of "a child is being beaten," as one version morphs into another, one might formulate the whole "complaint" situation in an even more oneiric, eerily neutral way, by leaving out any specific reference to the actors involved. For example:

There is a complaint against psychoanalysis.

As in a Kafka novel or a Bergmanesque existential melodrama, the nature and origin of the complaint are indeterminate. It could be coming from the patient, but it could also be from the analyst as well. In a certain sense, as Freud originally experienced it, the complaint comes from society. But the accusatory and persecutory themes remain constant, whichever way the elements of this bad dream are played out.

In our traditional way of limning such narratives, the first part—that the patient has a complaint about psychoanalysis; or, more fundamentally, that *there is* a complaint against psychoanalysis—is glossed over. What we are attuned to hear and what we are more willing to address directly is the patient's expression of that complaint in terms of sexuality, regardless how it arises. The complaint, made public, may even be that the analyst failed to satisfy the patient's sexual demand (see, for example, Heyward, 1993). In any case, the analyst either fails to respond to the patient's sexual demand in a satisfying way (e.g. the transference interpretations don't work), or the analyst responds in a literally sexual way toward the patient. In the first instance, we write off the patient's complaint as unresolved transference. (In such cases, colleagues may also write off the analyst's search for peer assistance and guidance in the same way, by making the argument, "What you are dealing with, difficult though it is, is really just the patient's sexualized transference. Don't worry about your own feelings, they're just countertransference. Keep analysing the transference.") In the second instance, where the analyst is found to be at fault, we use the fact that the analyst and patient *did* engage in a sexual relationship, which becomes a convenient fact to achieve a kind of secondary gain: it helps to narrow the patient's complaint down to the measurable instance of an individual analyst's overt conduct. In other words, if the patient has a complaint (or there *is* a complaint), we are willing to hear it to the extent that it refers to a sexual transgression. And we frame this not merely as a violation of the patient's trust, but more crucially for our sense of authority, we see it is as a violation of psychoanalysis itself. As Gentile (Harris & Gentile, 2019, p. 115) remarks: "The boundary, not the patient, was violated." Even in the case of "wild analysis," Freud (1910, p. 227) felt that the harm done is not so much to the patient as to the profession. (This is another way that we mimic retributive law: charges are always brought in the name of the State, not the victims.) Claims about the sexual nature of the malpractice may be entirely true, of course—but they are not necessarily the whole truth. The patient-victim may be saying all kinds of other things that we screen out, or set aside, or simply do not hear. The issue is not that we can ever know the whole truth, however; it is that when we train our ears to hear only the sexual part of it, we may fail to elicit, and perhaps never learn, what may be larger complaints against psychoanalysis, or the analyst.

We also fail to elicit, it should be noted, something that is undeniably within us all: that the analyst also has a complaint against psychoanalysis. We think we know all about this, of course, just as we "know," in another one of our pre-emptive fantasies, that everybody "hates" psychoanalysis because it threatens us all, analyst and society alike, with the "truth." (We talk about this a lot because it makes us feel important.) But this rationalization usually ends the discussion about complaints before it even starts. We are only just beginning to acknowledge that every analyst inherits a history of psychic pain and dislocation descending from generations of other analysts (Levin, 2014). Every analyst (with the possible exception of a few "contemporaries") has submitted to arduous "training" in a hierarchized, frequently highly authoritarian and elitist institution. Most analysts will have suffered the indignities and confusions of the training analyst system, which inevitably compromises the personal analysis and creates what Kernberg (1986) has described as a "radioactive" atmosphere. (It is not so long ago that training analysts "reported" on their candidate analysands to training committees and some (e.g. Britton, 2003) still believe this is necessary.) Surely there must be a long list of grievances that analysts privately harbor against their own profession; but there exists virtually no forum, no avenue, to address them in the psychoanalytic profession. Is it any wonder that so many of us "act out"?

To argue that we have been narrowing down the patient's and the analyst's complaints against psychoanalysis to illicit sexual actions is not to deny that sexual boundary violations are among the very most serious forms of ethical violation. We are certainly justified in assuming that the focus on sexual misconduct is an inevitable by-product of the catalytic role of sexuality in the human psyche—it is indeed a kind of proof in itself of the central importance of psychosexuality, which (as Dimen, 1999 was tireless in pointing out) is now often challenged within the profession. But to rest the argument on this consideration would be an over-simplification. A concomitant explanation for the ethical preoccupation with sexuality might be that it is simply convenient—it bifurcates the "professional" from the "sexual" in a neat way by literalizing them both, while keeping everything individualized on the behavioral surface. The concept of a "sexual boundary violation" is expedient because it is relatively easy to define for purposes of adjudication—and that seems to be why it has so successfully galvanized the beleaguered professional community into an organized deontological stance. The anxiety about SBV easily trumps other more difficult questions that might arise, for example: the question whether psychoanalysis, culturally and historically, carries within itself an implicit sexual invitation—and what to do with (or about) that. Is it necessary for psychoanalysis to be so daring with "boundaries," and if so, can the public handle it? Rather than explore such questions out in the open, we have buried them in the implicit consensus that sexuality is not so much a force in its own right as a defense. More specifically, we have avoided the looming question whether the patient's sexual complaint bespeaks a deeper form of violation, and conceals a more diffuse potential for mispractice, what might be conceptualized as "narcisssistic boundary violation" (Levin, 2014; Levine, 2010)—an ongoing process of colonizing the patient's mind, which may very well take place in the absence of any sexual activity.

In my own experience, "narcissistic boundary violations" have done far more damage to my local psychoanalytic community, broadly defined, than sexual boundary violations per se. To be sure, there have been some egregious cases of SBV, a small minority involving rank serial predators and psychopaths. But in these cases, it is in my view always the institutional cover-up that does the worst damage (see Ruskin, 2011). Other less pathological instances of SBV in my community have been shocking and terribly disappointing, but not nearly as debilitating over the long run for the community as the insidiousness of power hungry narcissists who go unidentified and unpunished, despite evidence of colonizing candidate's minds in training analyses and using their power methodically to prevent social change within the profession (to mention the more routine forms of systemic ethical misbehavior and dissociation within the group).

Among ordinary patients and candidates alike, there will be many analysands for whom, as de Urtubey (2006) phrases it, "to give one-self over to hatred from a persecutor ... relieves narcissistic fear of being insignificant" (p. 122, translation mine). Given the inherently masochistic component of any process as demanding as psycho-analysis (for both patient and analyst), this formulation may be closer than we wish to the essence of what is sexually attractive to many patients about psychoanalysis: not so much the invitation to sexual intimacy, but its endless deferral, as a simultaneously hopeful and despairing repetition of the unconscious belief that one is des-tined to be the object of hatred and envy. The latter may very well be the paradigm of many "training" analyses. If the analyst is prone to enjoy receiving this type of masochistic transference, which is particularly appealing to narcissistic power mongers, then the opportunity for wholesale (and sometimes lifelong) colonization of the patient's mind (continuing long after the end of the training analysis) is optimal. In such cases, it might have been better for the patient if the analyst had merely "fucked up" the relationship, either through gross mismanagement of negative ("counter")-transference (Levin, 2014), or even just by having sex with the patient. After all, when the analyst is openly hostile, the patient may simply leave the analysis, rather than remaining seduced and stuck by the hate; if the analyst's hostility is expressed through sexual abuse of the patient, or of another patient, the patient may be empowered by the deonto-logical code into tragic self-awareness and painful growth (see for example, Burka, 2014). Either one of these alternatives might be preferable to the successfully cold, narcissistic exploitation of the patient's addiction to mental enslavement.

Addressing issues like these would require us to venture into more ambiguous and dangerous territory where not only psychoanalysts fear to tread. "Narcissistic" mispractice would be difficult to define, of course, and (here is the rub), it would be very hard to say exactly how it can be distinguished from the idea of the psychoanalytic pro-cess itself (whether or not there appears to be a good psychoanalytic "frame"). Thus we can see how, in the historically turbulent rela-tionship between psychoanalysis and the public, in which the public has a long record of complaints, a convenient unconscious social bargain may have been established, for secondary gain. "Whatever it

is that is wrong with you/us, we'll call it sex if you'll call it sex."
And so thus we have managed to transform the potential for SBV,
the maximum flashpoint of our socially ambiguous role, into an
apparently clear demarcation of our professionalism, our immunity,
and our claim to "sovereignty." In our current model of ethics, this
sovereignty is supposedly exempt from what Levinas (1998, p. 141)
called "the extraordinary everydayness of my responsibility for
other [persons]." Singling out the sexual aspect of mispractice, in
the way we now do, nicely distances psychoanalysis from its own
ambiguous origins and historical legacy. To focus exclusively on the
sexual aspect of the patient's complaint then has this signal advan-
tage of keeping discussion as far away as possible from the internally contentious nature of psychoanalysis itself.

More crucially, it helps to keep the discussion, as Dimen cogently
demonstrates, out of the psychoanalytic group, or on its margins,
whether by drowning it in "routine dissociation," or steering it into
rumor and gossip. In her essay, "Rotten Apples and Ambivalence,"
Dimen shows why it has been so difficult for us to do otherwise—
our narcissistically invested idea of psychoanalysis as something
good and lovable (ideal), something healing and growth-promoting,
is threatened. Our sense of professional identity is (temporarily)
shattered. We fear the breakdown of psychoanalysis, not realizing,
in Winnicott's (1974) sense, that the breakdown has already
occurred (Levin, 2016). Because we have laundered, or failed to
mentalize, the transgressive nature of our own origins, we experience
SBV as external to psychoanalysis, a form of alien pollution. We
turn one of our own into an outsider, inadvertently relegating the
victim to collateral damage, while sidestepping as much as possible
the grievous emotional impact on other analysts. This projection (or
group projective identification) onto an imaginary "outside" then
becomes the source of a heightened sense of persecution within the
profession, and the cycle continues.

Dimen's exploration of these problems strongly implies the need
for psychoanalysis to move away from the retributive model, toward
something approximating the idea of restorative justice (see Gentile,
this volume; Harris, this volume; Harris & Gentile, 2019). There is
reason to hope that such a move might actually have a preventive as
well as a healing effect (Levin, 2018), where education has failed

(Gabbard, 2017). But this would depend upon our ability to achieve something that still appears to most of us very difficult and risky (and which may be impossible in some cases): to acknowledge and maintain the transgressor's status as a member of the community; and to recognize the victim, in whatever way possible, as having a legitimate stake in the future of the psychoanalytic project.

Part II: social aspects of psycho-sexual boundary violation

In their contributions to the companion volume celebrating Muriel Dimen's work (Levin, 2021c), Celenza, Elise, Guralnik, Frosch, and Slochower, each in their special way, addressed the clinical importance of the analyst's need for self-care, and the factors (narcissism, omnipotent self-abnegation) that undermine it. As Harris (2009, 2014, and this volume) has made clear in a series of papers, the analyst's self-care is also pivotal in the relationship between private practice and the analytic community.

The theme of self-care is taken up in more detail in Part 2 of the present volume with Terry Davis' remarkable and unique first-hand account of committing a serious boundary violation, the harrowing process of professional ostracism that followed the official complaint against him, and his personally beneficial rehabilitation. It is worth reflecting on the fact that Davis' problems arose during the closing phase of a lengthy analysis, during what was for other reasons already a period of tremendous stress for the analyst. The dynamics of "termination" in psychoanalysis are notoriously difficult. Brian Bird, in his classic study of transference neurosis (1972), commented on the tendency for the ending of the analytic process to be fudged in some way: "[S]lurring over a rigorous termination seems understandable. As difficult as transference neurosis may be on the analyst at other times, this ending period, if rigorously carried out, simply has to be the period of his greatest emotional strain" (p. 287).

Terry Davis is the pseudonym of a successful and well-respected member of the analytic community with something to say that cannot in our current professional climate be communicated without a great deal of protective insulation, not only for the analyst, but also for the patient. "Rehabilitation in a boundary violation from the perspective of the transgressor" is a rare and valuable contribution to psychoanalysis by a person who came very close to being entirely excluded from its ranks. Davis concludes this narrative of analytic crisis and professional ordeal with a series of well-considered recommendations designed to help communities mitigate the inevitable fallout from ethical violations.

In her thoughtful chapter, also informed by difficult personal experiences, Adrienne Harris builds an argument for significant reform in the governance of the analytic world. Outlining the need to explore very different kinds of dialogic and deliberative procedures, Harris turns to non-Western models of restorative and reparative justice for inspiration. Foremost among her concerns is the issue of human vulnerability—a condition shared by all stakeholders in the analytic community, first the patient, but not last the analyst in ethical crisis.

> At the heart of my concerns is a deep sense that self-care is often repudiated and even mocked by people in our field … This tendency to omnipotent functioning, responding to almost limitless demand, with heightened validation of suffering, creates a serious fault line in many analytic character structures, whether or not a boundary violation occurs. We are poor at self-care.
>
> (This volume, Chapter 4, p. 72)

Echoing Muriel Dimen in her move to the first person plural, from "Eew" to "We" (Levin, 2021a), Harris suggests that self-care will not find a secure place in our system of values until we learn how to address it at the collective level.

In her important paper "Don't Tell Anyone," Joyce Slochower (2017; in Levin, 2021c) highlights the distorting effects in the group of the binding (but also double-binding) power of idealization. In this volume, Katie Gentile reinforces the wisdom of Slochower's moral insight in her chapter "When the Cat Guards the Canary." She maintains that a crucial step down from our addiction to lofty idealization of psychoanalysis (with its attendant dangers of institutionalized grandiosity and submissiveness) would be to acknowledge the risks and limitations of professional self-regulation. Since Freud's (1914) original call for the creation of a "headquarters" for self-governance, psychoanalysis has made

a tradition out of exaggerated claims to epistemological autonomy and moral independence. Gentile challenges this guild-like
ethos with arguments that have risen outside the discipline and
challenge its pretension to be, as Freud said of the ego, "master
in its own house." Drawing on her own innovative research and policy
development of bystander intervention on the university campus, Gentile sketches an entirely new approach to sexual boundary violations.
Chiming in with Harris, she shows how bystander intervention could
transform the ethical equation within psychoanalysis because it
"demands evil and goodness be held together within the bystander."
Like the other contributors to this volume, Gentile further unpacks
Dimen's insight that in order to develop a mature sense of ethical
responsibility for SBV, the "we" (identity) of psychoanalysis needs to
integrate the "Eew" (disgust for the other) in what Gentile calls "a
more viable ethical third."

Avgi Saketopoulou's chapter continues the discussion of boundary
trouble with yet another and perhaps even deeper challenge to the
sincerity of our ethics discourse: not only do we dissociate the problem of SBV, she argues; psychoanalysts as a group dissociate sexuality itself, and the analyst's embodied sexuality in particular. What
she describes as the defensive "desexualisation of the erotic countertransference" comes with a cost. The convention of downplaying
the *analyst's* sexual transference in the literature creates a kind of
negative hallucination in the group, leading to three forms of self-
deception: that sexual risk is *not* inherent in the analytic situation;
that psychoanalysts are *not normally* intensely fascinated by their
patients; and that when we do become conscious of powerful erotic
transference to a patient, we may be tempted to interpret these feelings as "more real" and therefore worthy of action. As Saketopoulou explains:

> If we can't bear to know that our work opens up the possibility
> that the analyst may develop enthralling erotic passions about
> her patient, how will we carry out the psychic labor involved in
> giving up our patients as possible romantic or sexual partners?

Saketopoulou suggests a further cost of this defensive desexualization
of psychoanalysis: collective disavowal "cultivates a dense nexus of

unspeakable erotic affect" in the group, ripening the conditions for scapegoating dynamics that may unconsciously trap certain vulnerable members of the analytic community. Drawing on personal experiences during the period of her analytic training, Saketopoulou explores these important themes with precise descriptions and startling insight.

Part III: locating the psycho-sexual boundary

With sometimes very different but interrelated arguments, the contributors to this section challenge the underlying foundation of ethical discourse in psychoanalysis. To use an analogy familiar in philosophical ontology, they find our efforts to address SBV comparable to changing the planks in a raft that is already far out to sea.

Steven Cooper confronts the dominant analytic terminology of "sexual boundary violations" directly. Whereas the concreteness of this term as it is currently used, with its air of precision and its cautionary undertones, have lent themselves well to the political needs of our ethics discourse over the past 30 years, the same qualities may be misleading and even undermining in the context of thinking about the psyche, the analytic relationship, or the therapeutic process. Cooper argues that psychoanalysis needs to make a conscious effort to reanimate the boundary concept, letting go its forensic baggage. Brilliantly, he redefines psychoanalysis as a "boundary *art*," as opposed to the boundary morality that it has sometimes become in recent decades. His chapter explores creative and playful aspects of psychoanalysis as a mutual process of discovering and/or creating boundaries, emphasizing their mutability, and their function as unnecessary constraints or necessary illusions. Writing from a clinical perspective, Cooper proposes a practicing ethic of "perverse carefulness," allowing us to experiment with psychic boundaries as freely as possible. Sexual action on the part of the analyst would simply be ruled out of psychoanalytic practice as serious "misconduct" and *not* as a defining psychological issue that forensically overdetermines all our other thinking about psychic boundaries.

From a different but complementary perspective, Stephen Hartman radicalizes the concept of boundary from inside the social scandal of liminality, indeterminacy, and abjection—the pre-representational substance of sexuality and meaning. Like Cooper, Hartman is interested in psychoanalytic language, and wants to play with this language, with what he describes as the deliberate intention to "destabilize the over-determined sense of our disciplinary jargon, in particular the phrase 'boundary violation'." Primarily through a fascinating and original way of re-reading Winnicott, and his concept of the infant's "imaginative elaboration of bodily experience," Hartman forges a new language that evokes the somatic but also profoundly semantic stirrings of the nascent psychic body in a relational field that differs from the dyadic models currently in vogue. Using multiple meanings of the word "rest," echoing the post-structuralist "remainder" and other discursive strategies designed to resist the totalization of analytic concepts, Hartman takes us behind "mind" into a meditation on the liminal area, the in-between, of a *mine*field prior to symbolization ... not yet embodied, not yet conscious," where with Dimen's help he finds "the movement among, toward, and away from desire." Brilliantly provocative, Hartman joins the analytic process with anthropological "field" work in a common transformational project, an invitation for the subject to inhabit a

> transitional or potential space in which it becomes possible for a *constitutive boundary violation* to occur—one that relocates the mind in terms of the rest—that is, in relation to everything that has been left over and out in the process of "emotional development".

In a sensitive reading of the fine line between nurturing, as opposed to appropriating, the analysand's desire, as described by Dimen (2011) in her memoir of analysis with Dr. O., Hartman reorganizes the discursive space of analytic boundary language. He suggests that analysis offers a particular kind of psychically liberating "boundary violation" (perhaps akin to Winnicott's ideas about the possibility of mentalizing environmental failure through protected regression to dependence). Yet such journeys into the *rest* can be "powerful and seductive," creating the danger of an "overvaluation of the analyst's command of the field," which sets the stage for the psychic tragedy of a 'boundary *mis*-violation'" such as Dimen experienced with her analyst's slip of the tongue, refracted through Hartman's own poignant clinical vignette of a bizarre incident involving the tongue of an AIDS patient.

Hartman's essay is also notable as a memoir of his experience of Muriel Dimen's psychoanalytic mentorship. In both theoretical and personal registers, he evokes her mind in vivid images—of the way her body moved, and moved him; and the uniqueness of her analytic style. For Hartman, Dimen always remains within the compass of practice, never "applying" psychoanalysis to anything else, and never "applying" anything else (anthropology, feminism) to psychoanalysis; yet somehow, as he shows, Dimen infuses her intensely personal analytic learning into "a deep and tenebrous unity"—keeping culture in mind.

Ann Pellegrini's playful and humorous exploration of Dimen's *Lapsus Linguae* rivals the skill and daring of Cooper and Hartman in rearranging the ethical planks on the psychoanalytic raft. If Cooper questions the "boundary" aspect of SBV, and Hartman the "violation" aspect, Pellegrini confronts the "sexual" aspect, challenging the very idea of sexuality "as the privileged thing analysts must not do with their patients." Her question is powerful because it gets under the thick skin of confident psychoanalytic self-assurance about sexuality. To paraphrase Freud's parable of the three Copernican revolutions: is psychoanalysis really the master in its own house of sexuality? Might psychoanalysis also be an abject servant in that house, an unwitting agent of larger and more powerful cultural discourses, as Foucault famously suggested? In response to these difficult questions, Pellegrini builds on Dimen's "provocative separation between Oedipus and the incest taboo." While Oedipus addresses the developmental task of distinguishing one's own desire from that of the parents, it is not congruent with all the cultural possibilities of desire, and thus not synonymous with a supposedly necessary and fixed sexual boundary that marks forever the domain of what is rationally prohibited in human society. Pellegrini outlines a vision alternative to "disciplinary psychoanalysis" in which "psychoanalysis is also or could also be a place where we (analysts and patients) get to practice creative un-knowing together, including creatively un-knowing what 'sex' is or does or could be." In this scenario, "psychoanalysis might even open up spaces of freedom, novel modes of becoming, of pleasure, of care, and of relating to self and others … to un-know who you thought you had to be." To paraphrase Foucault, one would do psychoanalysis "in order to become other than what one is," a disturbing paradox that speaks to Hartman's idea of the field worker as the curator of an optimal violation, as a way of accessing the "rest," which in Pellegrini's language "encourages rogue selves, fantastic experimentations, creative fictions."

In the concluding chapter of Part III, I offer some reflections on Muriel Dimen's unique and inspiring vision of psychoanalysis, the drama of psychoanalytic love and the love of psychoanalysis, under the shadow of the primal crime. This essay is guided by the intuition that Freud's abiding confusion over the "nature" of the urges that constitute or inflect human being—that is, its open-endedness, its ecological unpredictability, or what he called *Trieb*—offers a clue to psychoanalytic boundary trouble. Freud put his money down on sexuality, but he deepened his thinking to encompass sexuality in a larger overlapping human current so powerful that it causes blindness and even bloody-mindedness (even in psychoanalysis!) about sexuality: what we still conventionally call narcissism, which is not necessarily a pejorative term. (See Giesbrecht & Levin, 2012 for a fuller outline of this approach to narcissism as *Trieb*.) Hoping to identify some of the cultural origins of narcissistic dynamics in the institutional history of psychoanalysis, I have singled out the educational philosophy in Plato's *Republic* and the social contract as envisioned in the biblical *Book of Exodus*.

Part IV: psychoanalysis *Unendliche*

In the final section, "Losing our psychoanalytic virginity," this book concludes appropriately with Muriel Dimen's overview of the many issues addressed in it, in an interview conducted during the tragic closing months of her life.

Notes

1 While influenced by Bateson (1972), I am not here using the term "schismogenesis" in the sense of his cybernetic theory of negative and positive feedback loops in the social behavior of groups.
2 For an interesting discussion of the possible role of systematic murder in the bio-cultural evolution (and self-domestication) of early hominids and hunter gatherer societies, see Wrangham (2019). Like Freud in *Totem and Taboo* (1912), Wrangham sees control of the alpha male types as a significant factor in the ascendancy of "pro-active" as opposed to "reactive" aggression in the development of human social forms.

References

Bateson, G. (1972). *Steps to an ecology of mind: Collected essays in anthropology, psychiatry, evolution, and epistemology.* San Francisco, CA: Chandler.

Bird, B. (1972). Notes on transference: Universal phenomenon and hardest part of analysis. *Journal of the American Psychoanalytic Association,* 20: 267–301.

Breuer, J. & Freud, S. (1893–1895). Studies on hysteria. In J. Strachey (Ed. & Trans.), *The standard edition of the complete psychological works of Sigmund Freud* (vol. 2). London: Hogarth Press.

Britton, R. (2003). Confidentiality and training analyses. In C. Levin, A. Furlong, & M.K. O'Neil (Eds.), *Confidentiality: Ethical perspectives and clinical dilemmas* (pp. 109–112). Hillsdale, NJ: The Analytic Press.

Burka, J. (2014). A chorus of difference: Evolving from moral outrage to complexity and pluralism. In R.A. Deutsch (Ed.), *Traumatic ruptures: Abandonment and betrayal in the analytic relationship* (pp. 126–143). London and New York: Routledge.

de Urtubey, L. (2006). *Si l'analyste passe à l'acte.* Paris: Presses Universitaires de France.

Dimen, M. (1999). Between lust and libido: Sex, psychoanalysis, and the moment before. *Psychoanalytic Dialogues,* 9(4): 415–440.

Dimen, M. (2003). *Sexuality, intimacy, power.* Hillsdale, NJ: Analytic Press.

Dimen, M. (2005). Sexuality and suffering, or the Eew! Factor. *Studies in Gender and Sexuality,* 6: 1–18.

Dimen, M. (2011). *Lapsus linguae,* or a slip of the tongue? A sexual violation in an analytic treatment and its personal and theoretical aftermath. *Contemporary Psychoanalysis,* 47 (1): 35–79.

Dimen, M. (2014). Inside the revolution: Power, sex, and technique in Freud's "wild analysis". *Psychoanalytiuc Dialogues,* 24: 499–515.

Dimen, M. (2016). Rotten apples and ambivalence: Sexual boundary violations through a psychoculturral lens. *Journal of the American Psychoanalytic Association,* 64(2): 361–373.

Freud, S. (1905). Fragment of an analysis of a case of hysteria. In J. Strachey (Ed. & Trans.), *The standard edition of the complete psychological works of Sigmund Freud* (vol. 7, pp. 7–122). London: Hogarth Press.

Freud, S. (1910). "Wild" psycho-analysis. In J. Strachey (Ed. & Trans.), *The standard edition of the complete psychological works of Sigmund Freud* (vol. 11, pp. 219–227). London: Hogarth Press.

Freud, S. (1912). Totem and taboo. In J. Strachey (Ed. & Trans.), *The standard edition of the psychological works of Sigmund Freud* (vol. 13, pp. 1–162). London: Hogarth.

Freud, S. (1914). On the history of the psycho-analytic movement. In J. Strachey (Ed. & Trans.), *The standard edition of the complete psychological works of Sigmund Freud* (vol. 14, pp. 7–66). London: Hogarth.

Freud, S. (1919). "A child is being beaten": A contribution to the study of the origin of the sexual perversions. In J. Strachey (Ed. & Trans.), *The standard edition of the complete works of Sigmund Freud* (vol. 17, pp. 179–204). London: Hogarth.

Freud, S. (1939). Moses and monotheism: Three essays. In J. Strachey (Ed. & Trans.), *The standard edition of the complete psychological works of Sigmund Freud* (vol. 23, pp. 7–137). London: Hogarth.

Gabbard, G. (2017). Sexual boundary violations in psychoanalysis: A 30-year retrospective. *Psychoanalytic Psychology*, 34(2): 151–156.

Giesbrecht, H. & Levin, C. (2012). *Art in the offertorium: Narcissism, psychoanalysis, and cultural metaphysics*. New York: Rodopi.

Grosskurth, P. (1998). Psychoanalysis: A dysfunctional family? *Journal of Analytical Psychology*, 43(1): 87–95.

Harris, A. (2009). You must remember this. *Psychoanalytic Dialogues*, 19(1): 2–21.

Harris, A. (2014). Psychoanalytic process in the shadown of rupture: Clinical encounters with death, death mothers, and deadly mothers. In R. Deutsch (Ed.), *Traumatic ruptures: Abandonment and betrayal in the analytic relationship* (pp. 13–31). New York and London: Routledge.

Harris, A. & Gentile, K. (2019). Boundary violations, consent, the law, and the lawless. In P. Montagna & A. Harris (Eds.), *Psychoanalysis, law, and society* (pp. 108–122). London and New York: Routledge.

Heyward, C. (1993). *When boundaries betray us: Beyond illusions of what is ethical in therapy and life*. San Francisco, CA: Harper Collins.

Kernberg, O. (1986). Institutional problems of psychoanalytic education. *Journal of the American Psychoanalytic Association*, 34: 799–834.

Kerr, J. (1993). *A most dangerous method*. New York, NY: Knopf.

Levin, C. (2000). Le devenir d'une acivilization: La psychanalyse comme virtualité du corps primitif. In D. Scarfone (Ed.), *L'Avenir d'une désillusion* (pp. 99–117). Paris: Presses Universitaires de France.

Levin, C. (2014). Trauma as a way of life in a psychoanalytic institute. In R. Deutsch (Ed.), *Traumatic ruptures: Abandonment and betrayal in the analytic relationship* (pp. 176–196). New York and London: Routledge.

Levin, C. (2016). Fear of breakdown in the psychoanalytic group: Commentary on Dimen. *Journal of the American Psychoanalytic Association*, 64(2): 381–388.

Levin, C. (2018). Revisiting our consensus on sexual boundary violations: A clinical, historical, and metapsychological analysis of the primal crime. Paper presented to the Michigan Psychoanalytic Society, Farmington Hills, MI, November 29.

Levin, C. (2021a). Introduction: From "eew" to we: An overview of Muriel Dimen's contribution to psychoanalytic ethics. In C. Levin (Ed.) *Sexual boundary violations in psychoanalysis: Clinical perspectives on Muriel Dimen's concept of the "primal crime"* (pp. 1–22). London and New York: Routledge.

Levin, C. (2021b). Boundary trouble in the psychoanalytic republic: Reflections on Muriel Dimen's concept of the primal crime. *This volume* (pp. 191–217).

Levin, C. (Ed.). (2021c). *Sexual boundary violations in psychoanalysis: Clinical perspectives on Muriel Dimen's concept of the primal crime.* London and New York: Routledge.

Levinas, E. (1998). *Otherwise than being, or beyond essence.* Trans. A. Lingis. Pittsburgh: Duquesne University Press.

Levine, H. (2010). The sins of the fathers: Freud, narcissistic boundary violations, and their effects on the politics of psychoanalysis. *International Forum of Psychoanalysis*, 19: 43–50.

Maddox, B. (2006). *Freud's Wizard: The enigma of Ernest Jones.* London: John Murray.

Ross, J.M. (1995). The fate of relatives and colleagues in the aftermath of boundary violations. *Journal of the American Psychoanalytic Association*, 43: 959–961.

Ruskin, R. (2011). Sexual boundary violations in a senior training analyst: Impact on the individual and psychoanalytic society. *Canadian Journal of Psychoanalysis*, 19: 87–106.

Slochower, J. (2017). Don't tell anyone. *Psychoanalytic Psychology*, 34(2): 195–200. Reprinted in Levin, C. (Ed.), *Sexual boundary violations in psychoanalysis: Clinical perspectives on Muriel Dimen's concept of the "primal crime"* (pp. 195–200). London and New York: Routledge.

Sundelson, D. (2003). Outing the victim: Breaches of confidentiality in an ethics procedure. In C. Levin, et al., Eds., *Confidentiality: Ethical perspectives and clinical dilemmas* (pp. 183–198). Hillsdale, NJ: Analytic Press.

Winnicott, D.W. (1974). Fear of breakdown. *International Review of Psycho-Analysis*, 1: 103–107.

Wrangham, R. (2019). *The goodness paradox: The strange relationship between virtue and violence in human evolution.* New York: Pantheon.

Young-Bruehl, E. (1988). *Anna Freud: A biography.* New York: Summit books.

Collective responsibility for the primal crime

Chapter 2

Rotten apples and ambivalence

Sexual boundary violations through a psychocultural lens

Muriel Dimen

Sexual boundary violations ferry analysts and patients from thought to action, from the symbolic toward the materiality of life. They bring the outside in. Yes, they are enactments of fantasy. At the same time, though, sexual transgressions are workings of power and vehicles of culture. They evoke the social context for psychoanalysis, its rules, politics, and disciplinary power, its ethics committees, the legal systems that license and regulate training and clinicians, define and punish breaches of sexual boundaries by the licensed. Sexual boundary violations make trouble for any group. And they are a problem of the group too.

Most psychoanalytic thinking about this problem tends to take an inside view. I am going to do so too, but I am also going to view it from the outside in. Thinking as an anthropologist, I consider psychoanalysis an institution that, like any other social unit, has a structure, history, rules, and beliefs. Since I am, of course, an insider, I can in no way claim objectivity. Nor would I want to. But my frame in this paper is different: a multiperspectival approach to this enigma, a position I am naturally inclined to take since in fact I approach sexual boundary violations in several capacities: psychoanalyst, anthropologist, whistle-blower.

I am suggesting that the phenomenon of sexual transgression between analyst and patient is insufficiently addressed as long as it is deemed to be exclusively psychological. Since it is also a social matter, as I am insisting, it needs to be understood by means of social as well as psychological concepts. And given that it is a group matter, it must be addressed by the group of which it is a property.

On this score, though, muteness seems to reign, in groups but also as a paradoxical way to hold the problem in mind. It is hard to have a thoughtful conversation about this particular aspect of group life. Sexual transgressions generate a great and contagious anxiety prompted by how they pollute and stigmatize anyone and anything in their vicinity.

The impulse to silence is fertile soil for intergenerational transmissions, that is, for the repetition of trauma. As one colleague said to me,

> If I know my colleague knows of a violation, that knowledge makes me so anxious about my beloved profession and makes me so fearful I will be tainted, that I want to put distance between me and that known knower even if that person never speaks of it to me.

Such terrors render sexual boundary violations unmentalizable, a hush that welcomes action as the only form of speech available. In other words, don't ask, don't tell, just enact. And so we come full, vicious circle. Breaking into it, I am saying, depends on thinking socially as well as psychologically.

I am quite taken with the phrase "the privatization of damage," by which the Latin American Institute for Mental Health and Human Rights (ILAS) aims to conceptualize how therapists might work with patients traumatized by the Pinochet regime in Chile. As I hear this motto, it calls into question the conventional psychoanalytic view that ascribes suffering only to interior processes and reduces political reference to a defense. Power structures, ILAS contends, must be regarded as an independent cause of psychic difficulty and trauma. The pain and anguish they occasion are a shared group concern, a public concern, and must be taken up as such.

Implicitly, then, ILAS's phrase indicates the way psychoanalysis tends to erase the cultural roots of individual difficulty. When it comes to sexual transgressions, for example, analysts, in keeping with their expertise, have historically preferred to focus on the unique individuality of suffering: perpetrators are ill, patients are seductive, exceptions occur, apples rot, throw them out. By the same token, familiar methods of the sort found in daily, noninstitutional group life are used to eliminate the disturbance: perpetrators are excommunicated, victims discredited or pitied, whistle-blowers isolated, apples tossed.

Yet thinking socially can partner with thinking psychically. One sort of social thought has to do with how groups preserve themselves. Every group, large or small, has a set of mechanisms that function to help it stay as it is, to maintain its institutions and beliefs and customs and power structures unchanged. Chief among these are ways of knowing and unknowing that discourage critical reflection on the group's fundamental premises, whether manifest or implicit. Here I would class the unspeakability of sexual boundary violations. Such an institutionalized shared disinclination—whether we would call it unconscious or unthoughtknown—functions to preserve the group's standing as a good object, but interferes with thinking about its problems and flaws: in this case, the phenomenon of sexual boundary violations. What will make such critical thought possible, I suggest, is to acknowledge ambivalence about the group, which itself hinges on some grasp of this phenomenon's place in psychoanalysis as a social institution.

The folk theory of sexual boundary violations

I want to highlight the efforts to understand and treat sexual boundary violators that have preceded mine and on which I build. This ongoing original research and theorization regarding the narcissistic pathology of serial predators (see, e.g., Gabbard, 1989) and the lovesick one-time offender (Celenza and Gabbard, 2003; Celenza, 2007) provide a remarkably sound foundation for further thought. However, this crucial work needs a more complex intellectual context. Our current discourse is what one might call a folk theory, captured in the saying "One rotten apple spoils the barrel." There's nothing wrong with the other apples. They are good. It's just that one susceptible apple has contracted those nasty mold spores that will travel to and ruin the others.

Guided by this folk wisdom, psychoanalysis repeatedly pitches the bad apple, only to find that, lo and behold, another rots.

Various responses to this repetitiousness are possible. One is to think, rightly, that we have not reached the bottom of the matter, whether you call it pathology, crime, felony, ethical breach, or transgression. Another is to wonder whether in fact all the apples in the barrel have it in them to spoil, which, as Gabbard observes, is also likely the case. A third, my point here, is that maybe we need to check out the barrel or, to follow Bion, the container itself.

For the aphorism I have chosen as a guide is a bit ambiguous: does the rotten apple spoil only the other apples, or is it thought to spoil the container too? It could be that one reason for chucking the bad apples over and over again is to safeguard the container that is psychoanalysis itself. Here might be one of those social functions performed by individual acts that together amount to another, unconsciously collective way of keeping the social unit just the way it always was. Since there's nothing wrong with the barrel, goes the premise, all that needs to be done is to eliminate the apple. But this solution invites a question: is the container endangered by the apple's mold spores, or does it also generate rot on its own?

It's my intent not to throw out the rotten-apple theory but rather to recycle it. So in this paper I am risking a mix of psychoanalytic and cultural ideas in order to advance a common concern: we have an institutional problem on our hands that requires collective thought because it exceeds any single analyst and any single patient, and exists at a level that cannot be reached by psychotherapy, supervision, rehabilitation, rules, New Year's resolutions, or even the buddy system that some psychoanalytic communities have adopted so that analysts may keep each other on track.

Psychoanalysis as a sexual field: beta elements and—K

For starters, consider psychoanalysis as a sexual field, "a matrix of sexual meanings, discourses, and practices embedded in social institutions [linked] to individual sexual scripts" (Green, 2014, p. 10). It is, however, an odd sexual field, for its brand is not a recognized practice like heterosexuality or barebacking. Rather, its brand is no-sex. "Psychoanalysis," quips Adam Phillips, "is about what two people can say to each other if they agree not to have sex" (Bersani & Phillips, 2008, p. 1). Don't even think about it, analysts double-bindingly tell patients. Open yourself to your desire and of course you will want sex with me, but do not imagine it will ever materialize, a prohibition that of course incites the forbidden longing. Don't get my irony wrong: this injunction is necessary, but it's also crazy-making. Or, better, it has interesting sequelae.

The taboo on sex between analyst and patient is foundational to psychoanalysis. Carrying on the Hippocratic tradition, it substitutes the meeting of minds for the embrace of mucous membranes. It creates an absence that widens, even generates, potential space. The gap also functions, in my view, somewhat like Bion's "preconception" (1962), an unstatable expectation of something not yet formed, neither cognized nor cognizable, a placeholder for the possibility psychoanalysis potentiates. Insofar as this preconception is fundamental, its violation sends shudders right down to the DNA of the psychoanalytic edifice.

This alarm might be said to be in the realm of beta elements. Unthinkable, these tremors show up, as Bion proposes, in the form of projective identifications. "Why is she doing this to us?" asked one person after listening to me give a lecture on a sexual breach I'd experienced in analysis, making me wonder whether I was harmful and, if so, what harm I'd done. What is shaken to its very foundation by the revelation of sexual boundary violations is the container, but the whistle-blower is made into the problem instead. I do not take such a response personally. I do not blame or pathologize the hearer. I interpret it rather as a sign of a shared, elemental refusal,—K in the service of protecting the container (Bion, 1962). Yes, everyone "knows" sexual boundary violations occur. But this knowledge is somehow compartmentalized and one-dimensionalized. It is a truth in the head, not in bones and hearts.

When knowledge enters the bones, however, it is more dangerous. Thus do I read the hostility in the question—not an inquiry at all, it was an accusation as much as a complaint. Perhaps when a colleague is straightforward, the fact of sexual transgression begins to percolate through multiple registers of knowledge, entering the empathic space that allows shared thought. When it thus gets under the skin, however, it also excites hostility, much as someone shoving you on the subway inclines you to shove back. A retaliation for what is perceived as an attack on the group's cherished belief—analyst and patient do not have sex—this hostility strikes back at the contagion that travels through the ether of empathy.

Psychoanalysis as a cultural institution: purity and pollution

Re-enter the rotten apple, which I now want to reframe as a cultural problem, that of pollution. Switching, then, from Bion to anthropology, I draw on Mary Douglas (1966), who in *Purity and Danger* argues that all human cultures create an opposition between the pure and the impure that functions to preserve culture by keeping order. The polarity arises, Douglas argues, in response to human life's inherent and culturally dysregulating untidiness: rotten apples being routine, the cultural problem is how to restore order when they show up.

Dirt is Douglas's signal example. Dirt is dangerous—impure—because, like all pollutants, it threatens to spoil everything: "Dirt [is] matter out of place" (p. 48). Dirt is "dirt" only relative to what is considered clean. Ubiquitous, it "is never a unique, isolated event." Rather, dirtiness and cleanliness are part of a system. "Dirt is the []by-product of a systematic ordering and classification of matter, []in so far as ordering involves rejecting inappropriate elements" (p. 48). Then we get to dirt's power to pollute, and the rules to undermine it. "Shoes are not dirty in themselves, but it is dirty to place them on the dining table" (p. 48). What is contaminating is not the item of clothing but its being in the wrong place; "food is not dirty in itself, but it is dirty to leave cooking utensils in the bedroom, or food bespattered on clothing ...." (p. 48). There is always dirt, but if each thing has its place and is kept in or returned to its place, purity will prevail.

When there are systems of classification, however, anomalies are inevitable. Not everything fits the either/or of binaries: think, for example, of how those people once called hermaphrodites, now intersex, confound the neat divide of male from female, and needed to be hidden away so their presence would not pollute everyone else. In anticipation of such problems, each culture has institutionalized solutions to restore order before disorder snowballs and poisons what is sacred, which is the group itself. In every culture are found ways to demarcate and separate the clean and the unclean—meat from milk, say, or beef from pork. Yes, beliefs and rituals dividing pure from impure foods may be shown to have salubrious effects.

That they do so, however, does not mean they cannot also function to maintain, by iteration, cultural health, that is, the identity, structure, and existence of the group, which also must be preserved at all costs.

By the same token, every culture has ways to repair the contamination caused by crossing such boundaries. There are usually very simple remedies for the effects of most mistakes. For example, if you accidentally put meat in the milk pot, you just re-kosher the pot. In rarer instances, though, transgressions are punished rather than remedied, the penalties cautioning against future occurrences, especially when it comes to sex. Some adulterers, for example, are branded forever (think Hester Prynne), sometimes they are excommunicated (Adam and Eve), and sometimes they are stoned to death or, like Anna Karenina, kill themselves. A measure of the group's sanctity, such actions, from the mundane to the catastrophic, function in the long run to maintain an ongoingly reliable structure for life: "rituals of purity and impurity create unity in experience," Douglas writes (p. 13). That such rules and practices of maintenance are also regulatory, serving as well to shore up a structure of power is not within Douglas's purview, though it should be within ours.

Seen in anthropological perspective, the proscription on sexual action between analyst and patient appears to play a role in maintaining the life of the institution. That this taboo is clinically and therapeutically crucial does not keep it from also serving a ritual and ideological function: as a premise, it is an emblem of the identity, integrity, and sanctity of psychoanalysis. Along with the requirement for personal analysis, it is one of the regulations by which psychoanalysis distinguishes itself among therapies. Its breach pollutes: sex out of place—sex in the consulting room—contaminates not only the parties to it or those nearby, but, I am suggesting, the entire institutional order of psychoanalysis.

Consider the way sexual boundary violations have traditionally been responded to, that is, by rituals of purification: the perpetrator is ill, so kick him out. Consider, too, how others are spoiled by the perpetrator's offense, like the victim, who, if she has participated in the sex, may be deemed seductive, so that her complaint becomes dismissible, and her perpetrator's act is expunged. Or take a bystander, like Sue von Baeyer of the San Francisco Center for Psychoanalysis. As she reported in a paper she presented at the Wounds of History conference in New York, after the news broke that her training analyst, Dan Greenson, had committed a sexual boundary violation, she experienced feeling tainted by the refusal of training analysts from her institute to take her into treatment (personal communication, February 2, 2016). A line between purity and danger is drawn between us, the clean, the good—and them: the dirty, impure, contagious.

Let me accept the charge: like our founder, I bring you the plague. But in what way? The questioner who asked, "Why is she doing this to us?" felt polluted by my story, because I refused to protect psychoanalysis from a necessary deep knowing: sexual transgressions perdure. In deprivatizing damage, my public discussion threatened the field's integration, purity, and unity: a kinsperson in the tribe we call psychoanalysis had violated a basic tenet, and, we are reminded, he wasn't unique. He has an estimable genealogy going back to Ferenczi, Jones, Stekel, Gross, and, of course, Jung, not to mention the many, many others lost in veils of secrecy and memory. No wonder sexual boundary violations belong to what Freud (1919) called "the uncanny ... that class of the frightening which leads back to what is known of old and long familiar" (p. 220). Such a lineage can only prompt the scary question: Is it something about psychoanalysis?

Is whatever keeps this phenomenon going connected to what keeps psychoanalysis going?

The vulnerability of psychoanalysis

Perpetrator, victim, and whistle-blower, their bodies marked by sexual boundary violations, recall the vulnerabilities of psychoanalysis itself. Analysts' and patients' bodies are carefully monitored, not only because of the Hippocratic oath but because, observes Douglas, the body's form, in particular its imperfectly closed borders, are quite apt for representing the aporias and incompletions of culture. By the same token, the body is quite suitable for rituals of purification. Psychoanalysis itself, a mortal institution populated by mortal human beings, has weaknesses. There is the rule against sex between doctor and patient that triggers the impulse to break it. There is desire, without which analysts cannot work, but which has no certain home in the work. There is the memory desire carries: sex tends to reignite unresolved incestuous frustrations and longings alongside quotidian but painful regrets about the failures and losses in love and sex. This incompletion intensifies the vulnerability to unrequited love that, under pressure of grief or tragedy (the lovesick analyst) or pathology (the serial or narcissistic predator) leap from representation to act, from Symbolic to Real.

The policing of analytic bodies takes on urgency for other reasons as well. It is not uncommon, says Douglas, for anxiety about the body to show up when a society is in trouble. Insofar as notions of purity and pollution and their associated rituals "express anxiety about the body's orifices, the sociological counterpart of this anxiety is a care to protect the political and cultural unity of a minority group" (p. 148). To the degree that bodies can represent the relation between parts of society, ideas about sexual danger in particular mirror patterns of hierarchy or symmetry found in the larger system (p. 14). In other words, anxiety about analysts' and patients' erotic orifices may be deeply implicated in the struggle of psychoanalysis for existence, which has been in question from the initial effort to establish the field, right up to the current battle to maintain its standing in public opinion and the marketplace. If purity is vital to social acceptability, then an unstained reputation is crucial. "Aren't you afraid you will hurt psychoanalysis?" asked a Canadian colleague about the paper I was writing. Already weakened, it needs perhaps to be in quarantine.

As the stain of stains, the violation of the analytic incest taboo may therefore be responsible for a task to which it is unsuited. If someone who happens to be an analyst and someone who happens to be a patient—of a different analyst—meet in a bar and go on to a sexual liaison, their encounter breaks no rule. Nor does their sexual relationship have the power to pollute: no boundaries having been drawn, none are violated. No order is disturbed, no pollution caused.

Between social and psychological: rotten apples and stigma

If what I have been saying so far about the social construction of sexual transgression and pollution holds any water, still it remains to think about how we get from cultural to personal experience. For this, I turn to Erving Goffman (1963), an ethnomethodologist who studied stigma, which he defined as "spoiled identity." If pollution threatens the whole social group, the threat of stigma divides it into two unequal parts, the discredited and the discreditable. Each of these has its own dilemma in the context of shared but tacit premises about normality, revealing stigma to be a regulatory practice in the operation of power.

These two groups are the inverse of each other. The discredited are those who carry the stigma of otherness: their differentness shows. Bodies marked by, say, the wrong skin color or a disfigurement or a disability, their lives are informed by the presumption that everyone knows about their discrediting feature. The discreditable, in contrast, are those whose stigma is neither known nor immediately perceptible. Only they themselves are aware of the potential discredit in which they live. These people are the normals, the majority who live in fear of being found out, of acquiring stigma.

Here is Goffman's remarkable insight: most people are discreditable. Most of the time, most people live with the fear of being outed for one or another potentially discrediting behavior or thought or thing—secret eating, for instance, or out-of-the-ordinary sexual practices (let alone fantasies about, say, having sex with a child or a patient), or politically incorrect beliefs, or maskable body parts that seem or are weird. Stigma is a set of social practices fueled by shame and a hierarchy of power that divides the acceptable from the unacceptable. As a system, it creates a truth out of a lie: the discreditable have something to hide, but their majority status renders them pure and normal.

In psychoanalysis, then, you could say that those who have not been involved in sexual boundary violations are the normals. This does not mean, however, that they have nothing to discredit them, just that they may not be discreditable by sexual transgression. But most have something in their lives that they don't want others to know. This discreditability is an unpleasant fact of life of which they are reminded when one of those with whom they identify—a colleague, or a colleague who is a friend—is stigmatized by connection to sexual transgression. This revelation in turn evokes everyone else's unvoiced terror of being outed and consequently discredited for a secret personal truth. Since, however, the discreditable cannot, or are not about to, get rid of their private dishonor, they prefer, by means of projection, to self-purify by eliminating those who cannot hide theirs. They erase the offender and the offended and the whistle-blower, and lo, the stigmatizing event that stains their beloved and precious profession never was.

To put it more generally, psychoanalytic life is burdened by a routine dissociation that is broken through when news of a sexual boundary violation breaks or when the phenomenon itself breaks into conversation. At such a moment, everyone in the group becomes stigmatized: the stigma carried by those involved in the sexual transgression travels to all the others as in a contagious process. But here is the truth: the stigma is, and has always been, latent in everyone. Perpetrator, victim, and whistleblower may be treated as Typhoid Marys, but in fact they are catalysts, for they prompt the ordinarily dissociated knowledge of what is already there. The fear and attribution of contagion mask the certain, and discreditable, knowledge that all analysts are already polluted. As long as the routine presence of sexual boundary violations in psychoanalysis is dissociated, the field needs to live in fear of being discredited.

Sexual boundary violations and those immediately touched by them evoke the irony built into human culture. Purity and pollution are a system. Evoking one conjures the other. If, as you must, you insist on keeping things clean, you are re-creating, with each act of cleanliness, the notion of dirt. If you insist on the rule of no-sex, as you must, you are insisting on purity, which then reinforces the notion, and possibility, and lure, of sex and pollution. As you identify and try to eliminate that which is polluting, you are implicitly identifying and trying to value that which is pure.

Hatred, idealization, ambivalence

How do you do something about which you can do nothing? The risk of stigma constitutes a profound fault line in psychoanalysis, and it is one of the rigors that generates analysts' hatred of their discipline. This hatred, argues von Baeyer, is a cause of sexual boundary violations themselves. Drawing on literature arguing various aspects of this thesis, she wonders if some aspect of sexual boundary violations may not be about "disavowed aggression [that] gets split-off and works insidiously as a hatred of psychoanalysis, ... the law, ... the principles that make psychoanalysis possible" (von Baeyer, 2013, p. 10). Convincingly, she details various dynamic and characterological processes, flaws, and illnesses leading to the expression of this hatred.

The problem, though, is not that we hate psychoanalysis but that we may not hate it. Let me explain. What von Baeyer does not illuminate is the phenomenon's systemic nature: however much individual pathology destroys a given analytic pair's capacity to think, which would normally keep sexual desire in the realm of representation and not in action, this approach does not shed any more light on sexual boundary violation as a recurrent problem of the group. For example, it does not explain the runaway anxiety that impels the normals, the discreditable, to act without thinking and eject the stigmatized and discredited.

I am about to go out on a limb here. So let me bring Winnicott along with me. Like him, I love psychoanalysis. But remember what he was brave enough to say in "Hate in the Countertransference" (1958): hatred is a routine, discreditable aspect of the work. The guilty are not the only ones who hate psychoanalysis, even if, in acting out, they act on that hatred in ways that, as Gabbard has noted, may incite envy and retaliation. Winnicott told us those eighteen reasons mothers hate their babies to illustrate why analysts hate their patients and, I am adding, their work. Nor will I detail the economic instability, the endlessly deferred and inconsistent personal gratification, the disciplinary hierarchies—where there's power, there will be hate—and the mental labor so layered and intricate you often cannot even remember who and where you are. I want to get to Winnicott's intent that we incorporate the hatred with our love for our patients, our work, ourselves; that analysts, like mothers, need thus to take on the ambivalence that is the core of our psychoanalytic heritage.

However, in regard to psychoanalysis itself, this stance feels as hard to hold as it is to achieve. It's one thing to diagnose the incestuous failures of the rotten apple who lets her destructiveness rip. And it's another to understand that the social body of psychoanalysis, like our unconscious development, seems to demand an idealization that is necessarily unstable. While Douglas, following Durkheim, says that the group is sacred, psychoanalysis calls it idealization. Whatever term you use, it does not admit of hatred. According to both institutional rules of purity and the unconscious need to idealize, psychoanalysis merits only love.

It is as though the psychoanalytic body is too fragile to bear hatred. As if it is so vulnerable to contamination and stigma that it cannot withstand searching inquiry into its inevitable flaws—for example, the nuttiness of a sexual field defined by a ban on sex. Could it be that the prohibition on institutional hatred also issues from the unresolved idealization of our elders that is built into the processes of training analysis and supervision and that maintain the profession's hierarchical structures? Maybe these ordinary parts of the psychoanalytic institution are the most palpable manifestation of an intergenerationally transmitted idealization that rolls all the way back to our totemic ancestor, the patriarch of the primal psychoanalytic horde, the one who analyzed the analytic great-grandparent of anyone who analyzed you. But where there's idealization, there is hatred, and therefore pollution.

Psychoanalysis, like any institution, entails endless rituals of purification, ongoing acts of idealization. Every conference, for example, must end with an affirmation of the discipline's absolute value. So must every paper, including, perhaps, this one. If you participate in these obligatory acts of purification, though, you also have a hard time thinking about the pollution that requires remedy, for example, about sexual boundary violations, because then you have to think endemic impurity, fault lines, stigma. How, given this stricture, is it possible to sustain ambivalence for anything, a posture that is necessary in order that neither hate nor love manifest as action, in order to maintain an atmosphere of K?

Thinking and knowing at all levels, in heart and mind and bones, inside and together, is necessary in order to reduce the incidence of apple rot. To think about anything in this full way, however, you need to hold it in ambivalence: maybe it's good, maybe it's bad. You need a critical faculty, to entertain skepticism about the thing, the work, the institution whose perfection is so unstable. It's not hatred of psychoanalysis that's the problem. It's the difficulty of ambivalence about it.

This is perhaps another way of saying that my concern is to move sexual boundary violations into the realm of K, to transform our responses to them into alpha elements.

References

Bersani, L. & Phillips, A. (2008). *Intimacies*. Chicago, IL: University of Chicago Press.

Bion, W.R. (1962). *Learning from experience*. London: Karnac Books, 1984.

Celenza, A. (2007). *Sexual boundary violations: Therapeutic, supervisory, academic contexts*. Lanham, MD: Aronson.

Celenza, A. & Gabbard, G.O. (2003). Analysts who commit sexual boundary violations: A lost cause? *Journal of the American Psychoanalytic Association*, 51:617–636.

Douglas, M. (1966). *Purity and danger: An analysis of concepts of pollution and taboo*. London: Penguin Books.

Freud, S. (1919). The uncanny. In J. Strachey (Ed. & Trans.), *The standard edition of the complete psychological works of Sigmund Freud* (vol. 17, pp. 217–256). London: Hogarth Press.

Gabbard, G.O. (Ed.). (1989). *Sexual exploitation in professional relationships*. Washington, DC: American Psychiatric Press.

Goffman, E. (1963). *Stigma: Notes on the management of spoiled identity*. Englewood Cliffs, NJ: Prentice-Hall.

Green, A.I. (2014). *Sexual fields: Toward a sociology of collective sexual life*. Chicago, IL: University of Chicago Press.

von Baeyer, S. (2013). Sexual boundary violations: A hatred of psychoanalysis. Paper presented at the Wounds of History conference, New York, March 1–3.

Winnicott, D.W. (1958). Hate in the counter-transference. In *Collected papers: Through paediatrics to psycho-analysis*. New York: Basic Books.

Part II

Social aspects of psycho-sexual boundary violations

Chapter 3

Rehabilitation in a boundary violation from the perspective of the transgressor

Terry Davis

I come to this topic because of my own experience as the guilty party in a boundary violation. As upsetting as this experience was, certainly for the analysand, as well as the other members of the analytic community, some of my other patients and myself, I am hopeful that my internal investigation and soul-searching may shed some light on this perplexing and troublesome subject. It is indeed unusual that a contribution to the analytic literature would concern itself mainly with an examination of the analyst's dysfunctional behavior when it is ordinarily the case that patients are the subjects of discussion. I have to confess that I do not come to this task easily. However, I believe that it is important that I, as an analyst who transgressed boundaries and learned a good deal in the process, write about this issue.

The boundary violation

I am heavily constrained in this discussion because of my concern for the patient's confidentiality. Therefore, I will not talk about the patient's involvement in the process nor give a detailed description of the process, even from my side, except in a heavily disguised manner. In addition, in order to protect the privacy of the patient, some of the description of what transpired is purposely omitted, distorted or left vague. In discussing what I experienced I want to make it clear that I am not talking about the patient but, rather, my experience as it was filtered through my psyche. Because of this, my decision to leave the patient out of my description of the process greatly restricts what I can say. Details in context would of necessity draw the patient into the discussion. On the other hand, although leaving the patient out of the discussion is a handicap, it may contribute to clarity of focus on my dysfunctional countertransference, and unapparent motives for my behavior.

In addition, I suspect that even if I were able to provide a detailed account of what transpired it would still be through my filtration of how it occurred. Presenting a narrative of exactly what transpired would invite speculations about different narratives. With that in mind I am leaving the sufficient statement that I take full responsibility for having violated the boundaries. Although the "devil is in the details," my fault is self-identified and it does not require full exposition to find the "devil." By focussing on the details of the narrative rather than accepting my acknowledgement that I committed a boundary violation the issue could become rerouted to questions of veracity. This is highly relevant since an often-adopted response to the problem of boundary violations is reductionistic – that the analyst who has engaged in a boundary violation is deficient in character. Such a simple explanation protects other analysts who learn of the boundary violation from struggling with the complexities of the phenomenon. Therefore, although it is not the primary reason for my not going into the details (the primary reason being protecting the patient's privacy), I am electing to avoid engagement in such a discourse altogether and instead focus on the essential issue of my experience as the guilty party in a boundary violation.

The violation consisted of inappropriate self-disclosures, some of which were of a romantic nature, which I made in the end phase of a long analysis, and in engaging in post-analytic meetings with the patient. Although it was not a case of doctor-patient sex, my behavior was clearly improper. The essential transgression was that my personal needs took precedence over the patient's reasonable expectation of being analyzed.

During the early years of patient A.'s analysis, I had become more fragile than usual due to circumstances in my personal life. This led to my being sensitive to criticism and I began to feel like I was walking on eggshells, especially with this patient. The patient knew nothing of this. But, as a result, I frequently found myself feeling defensive with A. Essentially, my neurotic fear was that the patient would be critical and devaluing. Nonetheless, the analysis progressed and I had the distinct impression that A. showed improvement with the analysis. The defensiveness that I felt related to my difficulties, I only came to understand better after the relationship ended.

The boundary violation began during the last year and a half of the analysis with my disclosing personal information about my life, which I had not done in the previous years of the analysis, nor with any other patient previously. In response to my perception that the patient could feel left out of my life, I decided to tell A. some personal information about myself. The slippery slope continued gradually over time with more self-disclosures as a result of undue pressures on me in my personal life. Termination with this patient became difficult for me so I decided for us to meet after we finished the analysis in a more personal context. The self-disclosures resumed during our post-analytic meetings. There was a major contributory event in my personal and professional life at the time that the boundary violation began. I became obsessed with my personal and professional crisis. The crisis affected my partners and me and although I took a proactive position to solve the problem, I felt, at times, isolated because of their relative passivity, leaving me alone to address the issue.

My conscious reflections during the boundary violation

During the period of the boundary violation I was extremely confused and troubled. I was mortified by my behavior but felt unable to alter the situation. It is noteworthy that it is often reported that analysts who commit boundary violations rationalize their behavior as somehow therapeutic for the patient. The victims of the abuse say that the analyst refuses to discuss or explore why he or she is behaving in this inappropriate manner. The lack of exploration contributes to transforming feelings into action. In my situation this was not the case. I attempted to explore my behavior with the patient, with the rationale of helping the patient deal with it, which only led to increasing self-disclosures. I was aware that my behavior was not proper but I felt compelled to continue it for reasons I could not explain. At one point I read to A. the ethical standards for practitioners, although in part I was attempting to justify my behavior by saying that I hadn't crossed improper lines. I revealed a good deal about the stress and other personal matters, trying to find an explanation for my behavior. I felt and at one point told the patient that I did not believe that my self-disclosures were part of the treatment itself. I was specific that I thought my patient would have had a successful analysis if I had not personalized the treatment. I did tell A. and believed at the time that my being able to be more emotionally present rather than distant and detached was helpful. Mistakenly I said that it was something that "just happened" and therefore could not be overlooked and therefore needed to be explored. Without understanding what was transpiring I didn't realize that even the discussion of it was a continuation of the inappropriate relationship.

I was aware that I was afraid of disappointing the patient and imagined it would lead the patient to feel angry if A. felt toyed with or misled. In this respect I was afraid that once I had embarked on this path I would be seen as betraying A. if I unilaterally stopped my engagement in this behavior. My fantasy of A.'s impression of me took on unreasonable meaning for me. It was as if I was determined to have A. like me and not be critical. I also believed that the previous years of analysis had been helpful and I was overly invested (selfishly) in the treatment having a positive result as if that would rescue me from being the object of criticism. I came to believe that I had positive feelings for the patient, rather than see it as a defense, and in that way I did not believe that I was being misleading. I also believed that A. was mainly concerned with having a successful analysis and in this respect I felt guilty. Although A. did not in any way control or determine my behavior I felt as if I were at my patient's mercy: responsible for an untoward tragedy, responsible for A.'s happiness and unreasonably expecting to be good enough as an analyst to cure A. of the problems which brought A. to analysis. I also felt trapped, both in this relationship and with the external stress of my personal/professional situation. During most of this period I was depressed and felt hopeless that I would ever extricate myself from either situation.

The series of events following the filing of the complaint

It is difficult for me to explain the chronology of events without including my personal reactions. I want to make it clear that others were hurt by me and therefore in talking about what I suffered through it is not an appeal for pity as if I were the victim. But, I am not aware of others in my situation that have written about their experience. Unless I include my emotional experience I believe an important piece of understanding of the process in the rehabilitation of boundary violators will remain obscure. From what I have known of others, they simply disappear, never to be heard from. On rare occasions the disappearance is complete, ending their own life through suicide. The void that is created – no explanation of their experience – is often welcomed because the "problem" has gone away. But unfortunately no light is shed on this important piece of the dynamic.

When the complaint was made I was humiliated and frightened. The ethics committee of the local institute took many months in arriving at a decision. Part of the process was the evaluation by an expert in another city. It was recommended to start a rehabilitation program, which was agreed upon by the local organization that had received the complaint. The rehabilitation recommendation consisted of continuing my personal therapy for three years, supervision with an expert on boundaries, working with a mentor and being on probation. During the time that this was being considered there was a great deal of conflict within the local institute as some of the faculty and students were angered by that determination. There were false rumors that I had engaged in sex with patient A. As one student told me: "people want blood." It was an enormously upsetting experience. One of my friends advised me that the situation would be better if I simply resigned from my position in the institute. I decided to do that to help the local group and to relieve the enormous stress that my spouse and I were going through. I did this, and apologized for my behavior. But that was not the end.

Over the next two years there were new procedural challenges by those unhappy with the ruling, which eventually led to my being expelled from the local institute. My reputation was ruined and I constantly felt ostracized and isolated. The ruling triggered reviews and evaluations by other organizations, which needed to be answered, at great emotional and financial expense. The shame and guilt were devastating as well as the financial repercussions and fear for my future.

I received help from several sources. The two that were most important were the individual therapy and the supervision. I'll talk more about the therapy later. The supervision was crucial. My supervisor first evaluated me and all the documents to see if he felt I could be rehabilitated. After he decided to proceed I found him to be supportive and yet clear in defining objectives and boundaries. His understanding of the essential issues involved in my behavior paved the way for us to explore where my vulnerabilities lay. I purposely selected two challenging analytic patients and went through process notes to see how I dealt with and metabolized hostile elements to their transferences. Beyond the supervision itself, it was enormously helpful for me to again feel that I had the confidence to keep my balance, stay engaged and work productively. My guilt over my past behavior, coupled with the constant proceedings where my character had come into question, had terribly shaken my belief in myself. Were they right about my being deficient in character? Was I was even capable of functioning effectively as an analyst? Was I really a bad person as many believed, or was it neurotic issues that had affected me? In many respects, that was the most troubling aspect of the entire experience. More than anything else, the supervision was crucial in helping me to regain belief in myself. I also had the loving support of my spouse, children and friends. A few colleagues at the institute were secretly supportive and loyal. I also had colleagues from elsewhere who knew what had happened and were wonderfully supportive. The other supports were from the parent organization and licensing boards that reviewed the complaint and took a less punitive, measured response.

Therapy for the boundary violator

For a period of twelve months after the termination of A.'s analysis I was so ashamed of my behavior that I was resistant to get help. Though I was aware of my responsibility for initiating and involving myself with A., I began to feel trapped because I could not get out of the relationship without prompting a complaint. I wasn't ready to face that, even if it was the ethical thing to do. Moreover, I was still bewildered by my conflicted feelings towards A. I realized I had to get assistance for my personal confusion, distress, and to manage the ending of the relationship, including help in tolerating a complaint if that was what would occur. I then had trouble deciding on whom I would see. Our local professional community was small and it seemed inappropriate to consult with one of the senior people at my level since of necessity we met so often as a group. I was also ashamed of exposure to one of my peers even if it were confidential. I knew I needed extensive help and did not think it was feasible to see a therapist outside of our small community. I eventually found someone to see whom I respected.

I suspect that when I talk about the issues, those who would only want to believe that the problem must be a deficiency of character would view any description of the therapy process as a formulaic rationalization or, worse yet, as psychobabble. I have to insist, however, that they were not in the therapy and could not emotionally experience what it was like for me. I might also say that it is sad for analysts who should believe in the value of therapy to want to dismiss its efficacy because of a preconceived notion of what they believe the problem to be.

I began our consultations by confessing to my behavior. I also began to explore in depth the stressful personal situation that had contributed to my boundary violation. The therapist remained fairly non-judgemental and listened attentively. I was surprised by his understanding reaction because I felt so ashamed. With no intent of disclaiming personal responsibility for my behavior with A., in time I began to appreciate the full context of the picture in which my boundary violation occurred. I was able to begin connecting the specific issues that the stressful situation triggered and to relate them to the conflicts that I struggled with in relation to A. The unfolding of the unconscious issues was a gradual process, which had several layers. It took many months for the relevant themes to become clear to me.

Eventually, I was able to realize that the stress had taken a devastating toll.

Ultimately, over a period of years, that situation finally resolved. My professional partners who were similarly going through stress had become depressed and paralyzed in coping with the situation. I responded, on the contrary, in a proactive way. In the process I was hiding from how depressed and demoralized I felt. Because they relied on me to be upbeat I was unable to effectively deal with my own fears. In this respect I felt abandoned and alone. Their fears affected me while I tried to reassure them. As a result it was very difficult to put it out of my mind as I had continually obsessed about this personal crisis.

In time, I began to realize that I had become unable to tolerate any perceived dissatisfaction by A. I realized that I had been angry about what felt like unfair treatment, which we were receiving, and unaware of my anger at A. Of course I lost the perspective that as a patient A. could and would be angry at times, like any patient in analysis. Rather than confront my hostile feelings for A. (internally) I transformed it into positive feelings. Similarly, just like I wished I could control the external negative criticism, I tried to prevent A. from being critical by self-disclosing. In addition, I realized that I imagined that A. felt envious of my having a "perfect life" as if it were something hostile I was doing to A. By revealing my problems I was in effect telling A. not to be angry because there was nothing to envy.

Later, in the course of my personal therapy, I began to see that I had become identified with A. Just as I imagined A. to be some-one who had been the victim of external events in A.'s own life, I saw myself as someone who was struggling against unfair treat-ment in the present. I admired what I perceived as A.'s strength and endurance and in this regard I became needy of A. – that by turning to A., I was hoping to find the strength to endure my own circum-stances. In this respect, I, as a survivor and hero, idealized A.

In exploring the childhood roots of my behavior with A., I came to realize that my personal narrative had never previously included seeing myself as a victim. Prior to the present circumstances I saw myself as fortunate in life. I had seen myself as self-reliant and cap-able. This led to my exploring how much self-deception was involved in this view of myself if I had become so needy now. In my personal therapy I explored my relationship to my mother. In my childhood my mother had been, at times, depressed and was often volatile. She saw herself as a victim of circumstance, mostly from a cruel father and as a result of poverty. As she complained about her circumstances, I responded by being her sympathetic listener and "therapist." I saw myself, in contrast to her, as fortunate and

therefore able to give freely. In my previous analysis I had extensively explored both the Oedipal roots and neurotic guilt that this
relationship with her generated. I now became aware of how it also
left me feeling deprived and how this was the perfect backdrop for
the current problems as they unfolded.

In my mind, I was once again the overindulgent "therapist" to both
A. and to my partners while feeling neglected with my own anxieties
and insecurities. By manifesting my neediness with A. I was also seeking to gratify those wishes, which I had previously been unable to
express. Further, because of the similarity to the situation with my
mother I was keeping my hostility towards A. hidden from myself.
With both my mother and the patient I had transformed my hostility
into positive feelings in order to protect them from my anger and
myself from my disappointment at not having had a caring woman to
attend to me. With A., however, the anger was manifested indirectly in
the harm I had done to A.'s analysis. The guilt over my neediness was
also manifested with the effects of my self-destructive behavior regarding my career and reputation. In the light of my professional success
I wondered, with some guidance, if I felt undeserving of the success,
which contributed to my self-sabotage.

After a complaint was filed my therapy took a different direction.
Both my therapist and I felt that many of the issues that led to my
boundary violation had been explored but that now I needed his
support to help deal with the fallout of the complaint. In this
regard the therapy was again helpful. As the protest by members of
the local community continued, and as the anger and mistrust of
me grew, I became increasingly marginalized. When I resigned my
position, I also apologized, with the hope that this would contribute
to healing for the members of the local Institute. I was mistaken, as
some members continued to be mistrustful and did not want me to
remain a member, even on probationary status.

In fairness to my analytic colleagues, I could understand how
they lost trust in me. Aside from my problems with the analytic
community, I was faced with a whole series of other consequences
as a result of the complaint being brought to several other venues.
Whatever stress I thought I had dealt with in the previous, now
resolved, personal situation, paled by comparison with the fallout
and consequences of this situation, although I knew I had brought

it on myself. However, the supportive aspect of the therapy was necessary just to help survive being the object of anger within the Institute and the cascading series of legal and practical ramifications emanating from the complaint.

Surprisingly, the stress of this situation afforded a new opportunity to work on some of the issues that my therapist and I thought were resolved in the previous psychotherapy. Aside from the guilt and shame I had felt and wrestled with in the first phase of my therapy, I now felt like the object of contempt by many in the therapeutic community. Previous to the boundary violation I had enjoyed a good reputation, which now seemed to be seriously damaged. On both fronts, my own self-regard and the esteem of others, I was in difficulty. In addition, because I no longer could be involved actively in the local group and had little contact with my former colleagues, I felt enormously isolated. The loss was profound since I had been so involved previously in both the institute and in the national organization.

At the deepest emotional level what was most painful was the anger and contempt from individuals with whom I had previously shared a mutually respectful relationship. Empathetically, I understood how hard it was for them to grasp that I could have behaved improperly, creating problems for the patient and the organization. I could understand their difficulty in trusting me again and why it was necessary for me to work earnestly in the rehabilitation program to regain their respect. Re-establishing my reputation with the very people with whom I had lost it was the hardest direction to pursue, but I knew it was the right thing to do. However, the continued proceedings and repeated attempts by some to reverse the decisions by the national organization and the licensing boards felt like a pursuit designed to have me expelled by both organizations or from professional practice altogether. The progress I had made in not worrying so much about the opinion of others was now sorely tested. It became difficult to know in the midst of my depression how much of my anxieties were realistic responses to a series of tragic outcomes and how much was a continued neurotic preoccupation with the opinion of others. To what extent was I internally separate enough that my self-esteem was not dependent upon the opinion of others? Who would get to define reality for me, my own observing ego and conscience, or the opinion of others who were working from their own realities? I did have the loving support of my family and friends (analysts and non-analysts) and the professional support I received from my analyst, supervisor and mentor. However, the same principle applied as with my detractors. My self-esteem needed to be independent of the opinion of others, be it positive or negative. The crisis became a catalyst for surveying the deepest level of my narcissism and issues of separation and individuation. As the work progressed, I realized that I could not seek the love of unloving others or go to extraordinary lengths to mitigate their hostility. At the end of the day I was accountable to myself. What opinions of me others held (positive or negative) emanated from their individual motivations and I could no longer rely on them to define my sense of who I was. I did not dismiss their concerns but, rather, I could respect these as their concerns. This insight was not only personally beneficial but also contributed to the clarity of my role as analyst. Empathy and intuition are only effective tools if the analyst has internalized (relatively) his or her own separateness.

Notwithstanding what I had gained, it had been a miserable, bitter and destructive journey. There was another loss I had to face which was also painful but necessary and useful. Previously, although consciously I knew better, I came to realize that I had idealized both psychoanalysis and psychoanalysts. Now I had to confront the reality that analysts were not necessarily able to divorce themselves from their own issues when they reacted to complex situations. They were not universally prudent and compassionate. Analysts were human, no better and no worse. Of course, I am including myself in this as well.

The question could fairly be asked: notwithstanding the conflicts that I have described, what really led me to in fact cross boundaries? It was not the case that I did not know where the lines were. In addition, I had always regarded myself as someone who maintained appropriate boundaries with patients. The ethics of the profession were not only something I knew about and subscribed to, but also something I fully believed in and felt was in the best interest of my patients. I did not have a secret belief that patients could be cured by the gratification of the analyst and with this patient in fact I believed that I had been very helpful in the previous six years of work when the work had been proper. Although it is tempting to think that regardless of the conflicts the answer lies in the existence of a basic selfishness, the answer may well lie elsewhere. I do believe that the combination of my unresolved issues, coupled with external circumstances, and a particular patient who could activate those conflicts, overwhelmed my ability to keep sight of what was most important.

Where matters stand now

It is many years since all of this happened. My professional life has continued and I enjoy a good practice with a mixture of psychotherapy and psychoanalysis. I have actively continued my involvement with the national organization. I became a member of another institute of the national organization and I have enjoyed a good relationship with the students and candidates at this institute. I decided to not try to get reinstated with the original institute for two reasons. To rephrase Groucho Marx: "I wouldn't want to be a member of a group that wouldn't want me as a member." From my end, it would be uncomfortable going through the process and I don't think I'd ever feel accepted. For the sake of the institute and patient A., who I understand is doing well and has risen in the ranks, I wouldn't want to stoke old wounds. The institute is now doing well and I am glad for both A. and the institute. The one question would be whether going through that process might help resolve past trauma, but the risks involved in disrupting all parties involved seems to me to be too great.

Recommendations for struggling therapists and organizations

Of course I am looking at this from my vantage point, having experienced first-hand all aspects of the situation. I am not suggesting that I have the answers since it is clearly tilted from the perspective of the therapist who has violated the ethics. So, what follows, are my impressions that emanate from that perspective.

1. If the culture towards boundary violators is rigidly hostile, it prevents therapists from getting help early in the slippery slope. Many of us may need supervision or therapy at times during a difficult phase of life or with a particularly challenging patient. But fear of humiliation, as in my case, may delay the period of time before an analyst seeks help. If our expectations are of

a punitive response, beyond our own natural shame and confusion, the delay can lead to further decay along the slippery slope. This is the reason that I have agreed to write this chapter with the hope that it can increase compassion and understanding. Without that the task of rehabilitation becomes ever more daunting.

2. It is more difficult for a senior or esteemed analyst to get help early on. It is the analyst's expectation at this stage in their career that they should be able to solve their own problems. Also, the shame is greater because it would be more understandable for a junior person to seek consultation. For a senior analyst to seek help the risk is greater. Automatically they would assume that in addition to anger and disappointment they would expect the other members of the group to feel betrayed by one they admired. Organizations responding to complaints should appreciate this factor. The culture of every institute should include the awareness that we need help and support throughout our lives – seniority does not prevent unconscious countertransference problems from occurring.

3. Certainly the victim, but also the transgressor, needs support after the complaint has been made. The investigation process goes on much too long (often many months), and during that time both parties should have an ombudsman keeping them minimally informed so that all of their fantasies of being ignored are kept at a minimum. I can speak for myself but I think it must be true for both parties that the fallout of the complaint and all of the misinformation can lead to an awful sense of isolation.

4. Regardless of the decisions that are reached, an active effort should be made to have some opportunity for the violator to apologize to the victim. That can only happen when the transgressor is in a place to take total responsibility. Sometimes the victim may be reluctant for various reasons: fear of the violator or fear, paradoxically, of diminishing the sense of injury, to his/her sense of entitlement to the injustice. However, remaining permanently in the "victim" role may not be in his/her long-term best interest.

5. There can be insensitivity to the victim with a misguided belief that they are partly responsible for what happened. It should always be understood that regardless of the circumstances it is the treater who is responsible for preserving the boundaries. That is a compassionate response. Similarly, the transgressor may have acted out of an internal problem and now be in serious trouble. To respond to the transgressor as someone in need of help would also be a compassionate response.

6. I was advised by a senior analyst to talk individually with different people upset with me. In retrospect I don't think it was good advice since my attempt to explain why I had acted as I had was only seen as defensive (which I'm sure in some way I was at the time).

7. People who have gotten into trouble need to believe that if they follow through responsibly on their rehabilitation that there is a professional life after. It is hard to believe that when one is in the midst of the endless proceedings, determinations and consequences. Also, since I treated several individuals in the mental health field, many of them learned about the complaint. Uniformly, when asked, I told them what it was about and took responsibility. Every such patient seemed to appreciate that and continued in treatment.

8. I am of the opinion that organizations need a great deal of guidance from larger overseeing bodies and outside consultants. In my case the licensing boards and the national professional organization more wholeheartedly supported rehabilitation than the local Institute. This is understandable, especially if the complainant is a member of the local Institute. The degree of injury is keenly felt locally and there can be a wish to rescue the victim from the violator. I also think that many in the local institute feel weary of the conflict and want the problem to simply vanish so that they can go about the important work that they do. That contributes to not supporting rehabilitation. When in the midst of a maelstrom it is hard to have an objective voice. Outside experts can see matters more clearly.

9. When the transgressor is first exposed for their behavior it should be expected that they would be defensive and frightened. It will take many months for him/her to metabolize what has

happened and to have some understanding of it. That would also include the ability to take full responsibility. It should not be assumed that because they are defensive at that time that they are automatically characterologically disturbed and not capable of rehabilitation.

10. Also, even if they have worked through important aspects of their problem they are now under attack. So much is at stake and the new situation is in itself traumatic. It should be expected that they would try to defend themselves, from the very serious repercussions. This is not the time that the evaluating organizations can have a clear perspective on how the transgressor really feels or their capacity for rehabilitation.

I believe that national professional organizations should publish a list of experts around the country who could help transgressors who are running into difficulty early on. It should be agreed that they would have the full protection of confidentiality. In that way they would have the ability to find someone outside their community who could guide them. It may be advantageous in some cases for this consultant to be someone who has been through the repercussions of a complaint and been rehabilitated. It may be less shameful for the transgressor and therefore more likely that they would seek help if they were to see someone who has been through the experience. Also, such a consultant may have good advice about how to navigate the myriad pitfalls awaiting them.

I acknowledge that I present all of this in a voice biased by my own experience. I am sorry to relay the personal trauma, since it is not an appeal for sympathy but rather a way of giving a human voice to what actually happens when one is exposed. I could have elected to not write this chapter since there is nothing to be gained for me personally any longer. But I did feel it is important to elaborate on some of the complexities of ethical boundary situations that are usually ignored. Also, we are in a profession dedicated to helping people and saving lives. We all agree that the well-being of the victim long-term is important in order to help him/her to resolve the trauma and have a successful life. The same should be true for the transgressor.

Chapter 4

Boundary violations as assaults on thinking

Consequences and remedies

Adrienne Harris

It is now (finally) axiomatic in writing about and conceptualizing boundary violations to notice the severity of the damage and the scope and range of who is damaged and how. The violation of trust, the attack on linking of past present and future, the self-critical worry that it is the analysand's judgment that was impaired, the huge and seemingly unending costs of splitting, the death of goodness very widely conceived: these outcomes occur at the individual and at the collective level.

A boundary violation is certainly an attack on the analysand who is victimized. It is also an attack on the community that has supported and often deeply esteemed the person committing the boundary violation (Pinsky, 2011). As someone in a community in which boundary violations have occurred, I think often that these acts were made out of a hatred of psychoanalysis, of its disciplines and demands, and of its practitioners. Whether this is the perpetrator's intention, I cannot say definitively, but it is my experience, as an engaged member of psychoanalytic communities large and small.

The irony and the ghastly truth, of course, is that there is no analytic community immune from boundary violations. Boundary violations were present in the earliest periods of our psychoanalytic history, both as the acts of serial offenders and single instances that appear to have been driven by some particular set of circumstances. So whatever conclusions or themes and processes one discerns in the current situation one can assume that these effects have leaked through a number of generations. This global and totalizing aspect of boundary violations adds to the terrible difficulties for community members in managing such events as they intrude into collective consciousness. We swim in poisoned waters.

I have to notice my own ambivalent moves to and away from the language of criminality. Victims, perpetrators, collateral damage, bystanders, communities' standards and well-being. I want to insist on this language throughout this paper and then finally try to find a new language to encompass the community tasks in reparation.

Incest and the primal scene

In 35 years of practice, I have had experiences with boundary violations in my communities, most of which follow a familiar path. I have had colleagues, some close, some more distant, all very revered and admired, accused of boundary violations. All took some steps to move away from the community, leave posts in institutions and community projects; in some cases they retired medical licenses. All these practices were believed to be acknowledgments of culpability, and strategies to avoid official censure. None of these individuals made any acknowledgment publicly of what had happened. I have no experience of someone expressing remorse and in most cases, there is simply a disappearance, in fact and in discourse, of the person who is believed or known to have committed a boundary violation. The imposition of silence is ubiquitous.

Perhaps paradoxically, silence in the communities and their subgroups are often fear-driven, built on the worries about lawsuits and a punishment of the community member who speaks out. I say paradoxically because it is the bystander who is fearing punishment, often from the accused person who will sue on the basis of harm to his/her reputation. As well, we are all very familiar with the antagonism socially to the whistle blower, the person who breaks silence. Dimen (2011) has written about this in the context of her ongoing experience of having spoken out and written about a boundary violation which she experienced.

I therefore speak as part of the collateral damage, a practitioner who feels that the practice, and the community of practitioners, and the theory itself are damaged by boundary violations. This damage has been with us from the beginning of psychoanalysis and its intergenerational effects we are just beginning to be able to see and assess. While we know many of the details and incidents that appear very frequently among the reports and accounts of early days in analysis, we don't always think about the long shadow of intergenerational effects that these early transgressions may have initiated. The long-term effects of boundary violations are part of the unspeakable history of this field, a history that threatens always to erupt and reinjure all of us.

I think the problems of silence and speech in the communities (micro and macro) are not merely a fear about litigation. When I reflect on the experience of discovering and assimilating an instance of a suspected boundary violation, I have always in some form or other had an experience of quite extreme cognitive and affective destabilization. It has taken different forms. I would feel that my upset itself was a problem, a symptom of something wrong with me. In extended discussions and conversations I would feel crazier and crazier. Who was the violator here? I think this worry surfaces in our fear of lawsuits. However real such fears are, they must also be driven by the unconscious guilt and terrors that the criminal is oneself.

As I do engage in more conversations and discussions about boundary violations, I see that my symptoms are ubiquitous. A colleague requesting some public forum for discussion and continuing to make the request when the initial query was ignored, was finally asked by a more senior colleague why she was so wrought up by this. The problem had migrated from perpetrator to bystander. Guilt was so contagious it could be acquired simply by a show of interest or concern.

Here, I think, we must pursue a psychoanalytic answer. Among other matters, a boundary violation breaks our western, first world version of the incest taboo, a taboo of near universality. Given transference and countertransference, we must experience the breaking of an absolutely indissolvable boundary between parent and child to be at the heart of a boundary violation in an analytic treatment. To the degree that a taboo always entails and even privileges anxiety about its breaking, the violence of incest within a community must destabilize everyone. Through processes of identification or projection, the surrounding people, close or far from the center of the crisis, must feel implicated. Every element or instance of erotic countertransference that has arisen in our practices or supervisions rises to haunt us.

We need not forget that we have unconscious elements that remain untamed and always partially unmanageable. How can we practice psychoanalysis without this understanding of everyone's vulnerability? I don't think I am exactly saying that anyone can commit a boundary violation but that with the alignment of various forces and circumstances, a risk, never entirely absent, may reach impossible levels. And most importantly, I am arguing that the vulnerability to anxieties about taboo breaches, even if such breaches never occur in an analyst's life and practice, create, in him or her, heightened levels of anxiety when something does occur in the community. This vulnerability is the by-product of the necessary agreement analysts make to work with uncertainty and to be able to notice and tolerate the ongoing mysteries of elements in the unconscious, particularly the erotic.

In communities, the silences and the silencing create the worst conditions for healing splits and sometimes fatal alienations. Institutes and communities have actually been destroyed by the appearance and mismanagement of boundary violations. Here I believe we find the potency and terror evoked by the primal scene.

When a boundary violation is uncovered, in print, or through communications within a community, a private door is thrown open, something unsavory and dangerous revealed. We feel excluded. We feel sick. We feel grateful if our analyst has been steady and containing. We fear that everything will be destroyed: reputations, livelihoods, communities. A tsunami threatens. In this mix there is both perception and fantasy.

The primal scene has been of interest in some theoretical endeavors more than others. Bionian and Kleinian, classical and modern, anchor development with a mature genital couple as a kind of structuring background. The system is potentiated by barriers, hierarchy, and exclusion, with its humiliating but also relieving features for the child. Aron (1995) argues for the solidly closed door as a necessity for the flourishing of fantasy.

It must be that the revelation of a boundary violation invokes both a breaking of the incest taboo and a dramatic, even violent plunge of all surrounding persons into the sight and reality of the primal scene. Guilt, but a guilt also linked to excitement, is at least one of the inevitable outcomes of simply being a bystander. Many people in analytic institutes have experiences and knowledge of boundary violations as an intergenerational problem. Whether carried as rumor or factual history, these phenomena make institutes unsafe. And unsafety is one of the derailers of thinking. Because legal issues often seem to force a collective silence, the mix of fantasy and reality in regard to the health or weakness of one's institutional home remains unanalyzable. We are often enjoined not to use the most important tools in our professional lives: introspection and relatedness.

-K: vulnerability and dissociation

Bion (1962, 1970) designated K to describe a function which he always saw as linking knower and known. He considered that such relational configurations could be characterized by L or H and he was also interested in how to describe what happened when the link with K failed and thought seemed adrift, either collectively or within the mind and being of one person.

I consider that my inability to remain coherent to myself, to be able to think and stay attached to my community and cohort, is connected to a number of psychic factors. The confusion of tongues, to call on Ferenczi, the muddle as to who is bad and who good, the strange contagion of sickness and badness, all seem part of the terrible collapse in functioning that befalls communities and individuals as they/we confront boundary violations. There is so often a strange mixture of gossip and furtive detective work. Conversations can be discreet or indiscreet as information streams both unchecked and at the same time blocked and secretive in the institutional communities where a boundary violation has occurred.

The struggle to think is what Dimen (2011) wrote about extensively, not only in the context of the treatment and what occurred there but in the aftermath of her speaking and writing. This has made me think of Ruth Stein's (2005) writing on the perverse pact and on perversion as lying, as upending reality, as living in quagmires of hatred and psychic violence. But I mean to think of this in all directions, perversity emanating from the community, from the boundary violator, from leaders and followers. It may also be that the victim's hatred feels perverse, feels forbidden and spoiling. I am deliberately trying to paint a picture of psychic wreckage whether in small groups or large, in the dyad at the center of the trauma or in conversations even with trusted others. We lose our way.

As I read and participate in the increasing and increasingly open and subtle writing on the complexity of transference and counter-transference entanglements (Davies, 1996; Aron, 2000; Harris, 2009; Katz, 2014), I feel that the struggles I am describing are acute when the issue at hand is boundary violations; but these problems arise at the level of the individual and of the group in many circumstances and situations. Illness, impasse, loss, vicissitudes of personal life at many stages of life and in many directions. In all these situations, including the impact of boundary violations at all levels in a community, we are hampered by two factors, one that is unchangeable, one that would be mutable if we had the will to do so. The factor that will be unchangeably difficult is the uncertainty endemic to clinical work. As the psychoanalytic century has rolled onwards, this has only gotten more severe. We do high stakes work in a dynamic field situation which will always have some degree of unpredictability.

The feature of our work which could change is the conversation and matrix of holding and talking that surrounds all of us. The habits and reflexes of the group, our institutes, our communities and sub-cultures, have failed in so many ways to provide real conditions of safety. Or perhaps one should say 'good enough safety'. These conditions arise when there is freedom to talk. Ironically, the domain of psychoanalysis, determined to create as much safety and freedom for the patient as is possible, has not been able to secure the safety of the analyst. Again, at its best such process would provide good enough safety, not perfection.

-K becomes a property of the group. But that paralysis of mindfulness and reflection may be intertwined with a fantastically and fantasy-laden set of pre-occupations among group members. When Bion thought about K, he always felt it to be K in relation; that is, that K was a function undertaken by one person in relation to another or others. The disruption of K in group process, what Goldberg (2008) has termed the disruption of communal dreaming, is replaced by fantasy constructions in which shame, degradation, envy, and a shattering of idealizations dominate. These states or fantasies, at individual and group levels, disturb the group's capacities to hold complexity and process events happening within the group. This may be one mechanism or set of mechanisms through which unprocessed experiences and feelings about boundary violations are unconsciously passed on intergenerationally in institutes.

At a recent Division 39 panel on boundary violations (Dimen, 2017; Jurist et al., 2017; Slochower, 2017, this volume) speakers addressed these community-wide conscious and unconscious forces. There is the role that idealization plays in protecting and then also wishing to dethrone revered analysts in a community who commit boundary violations. There are oedipal dynamics that inevitably influence and shape the stratification and hierarchies in institutes. Often there is a chosen student/candidate/analysand elevated to special and beloved status by a community leader. There is the lethal effect on group cohesion and functioning of secrets that elevate some and exclude others. Chosenness in a family, in a dyad, or in a group must lie on a spectrum of normal to pathological. There are inevitable differentials within groups at all levels, but the secret or revealed presence of boundary violations contaminates everyone. Feelings of jealousy, of exclusion, of rejection, tapping into very primitive states in all of us begin to create a hideous background to the community's efforts to think and proceed rationally. All this disrupts our capacity to think.

Hatred of psychoanalysis

As I noted in my introduction to this essay, in my experience of learning of a boundary violation, particularly when the person has stature in the field, I have always had the visceral and immediate thought that this comes from a hatred of psychoanalysis. I feel this personally and at a primitive level. Psychoanalysis has been attacked, a lethal blow dealt. It feels personal, it feels institutional. What I now suspect but have a hard time facing is that this hatred must also be mine and that in my projection of hatred onto the one doing a boundary violation, I rid myself of the troubling thoughts about this profession, this work, this inherent burden in being a psychoanalyst.

Why hatred? It may be one response to feeling burdened by ideal-izations: of patients or colleagues. It may be the underside of the discipline and (at times perhaps masochistic) requirements of the work. It may be a reaction to working always with fear and uncer-tainty. Hatred may be an occupational hazard of healing practices. And certainly, this would follow from Winnicott and others' atten-tion to the role of hatred in moral development, particularly as he wrote about maternal hatred. The mother hates the baby, Winnicott (1949) suggests, because of all she must do for her/him, all the sacri-fice and self-control this requires, the variability and often the impossibility of gratitude and reciprocity from the child. All these factors may enter our work and it can be hard, as Winnicott pro-poses, to see that hatred and love intermingle.

In the wake of learning about a boundary violation by a colleague, whether that colleague is close or distant, I think the bystander, the collateral damage, the group member may feel hateful and hated and the virulence of perhaps only semiconsciously under-stood aggression takes its toll on the individual and the group. The location(s) of aggression are unstable. For many analysts this may lead to a general constriction of imagination and affect, a thinning of countertransference and the tendency to live in treatments in a rather shallow stream.

The unmetabolized presence of hatred at individual and group levels clouds our capacity to think and to be willing to examine closely what has happened and what might emerge as the collective wisdom within the group. Here I mean by "group" many different groups: the profession, subgroups, theoretical orientations around which people group, institutes, training programs, clinics or sites of clinical practice. Groups, Bion teaches us, can fall ill, lose their pur-pose and task and become instead sites of splitting and alienation and much disavowed aggression. This fate of group process is per-haps nowhere in psychoanalysis more true than in settings where a boundary violation has occurred but its validity, meaning and impact are nowhere addressed or processed.

Gabbard and Lester (1995), and Celenza and Hilsenroth (1997), sug-gest that there are a range of experiences, a spectrum, of events and actions that go from boundary crossings to sexual boundary violations. Here we have to be prepared for individual differences in how this spectrum is parsed. For some people, the issue of a sexual boundary violation resides exclusively in a dyad where there is a patient under care. For others, violations arise wherever a power differential (teacher/student: supervisor/supervisee) is in play. Universities now have quite elaborated strictures on relationships that cross hierarchies, within that context. Most psychoanalytic institutes do not articulate policy on this matter, though there are many private views and consequences when such relationships appear or are suspected within a group (see also Gabbard & Peltz, 2001; Celenza, 2007).

There must also be quite careful considerations about the question of rehabilitation. While there is most usually a demonizing and exclusion of a known and identified or acknowledged boundary violator, there is a much less articulated process of repair and rehabilitation. Some of this difficulty in articulating policies about reparation or reconciliation may speak to the unconscious forces of hatred and sadistic pleasure at triumph and punishment and the attendant fears and confusions that such forces of exclusion provoke (see Davis, this volume).

What is clear from any discussions, public or private, about the impact of boundary violations upon groups and their members, is that silence is lethal. Almost any attempt to genuinely address people's fears and angers lessens the force of hatred and -K. These internal forces of dissociation and evacuation limit our ability to think and to think together. Exploration and discussion enable a return to some interrelatedness in groups. Such a process can result in significantly more ability to think and hold complexity. How is it that what we expect and hope for in our patients is so hard to achieve among ourselves in times of crisis?

For about eighteen months, a group of psychoanalysts, from different institutes within our city (New York) came together to work on a conference on boundary violations, driven to create an independent structure in which to engage with boundary violations. We were inspired by and intending to focus on Muriel Dimen's work. We failed and disbanded with some faint and perhaps naïve hope to reconstitute. Leadership of the conference had shifted around. It seemed for a while the conference was homeless, enjoined or impossible in several settings for reasons that always seemed simultaneously clear-cut and opaque.

The process of discussion was powerful. We worked towards a vision of a conference in which we avoided demonized others, kept the contradictions in the room. As one of the co-leaders coming into the process mid-way, I managed to enact many of the pitfalls of work on this matter; forgetting, erasing, fearing real and imaginary dangers. The focus on Muriel Dimen's work got lost or sidetracked and marginalized, a process in which I was certainly implicated. The prominence we gave to sex frightened off at least one of our intended speakers.

The collapse of the committee and the conference idea came on the heels, I would say, of fears and a sense of danger that swamped us. Perhaps some of our plans and ideas were too freewheeling, too provocative. Lawyers, asked to weigh in on various forms of dialogue and deliberative process we were designing, voiced alarm. And as always with lawyers, one has to wonder, were they correct, overly lawyerly, or merely the repository of our terrors. Fantasies of lawsuits, damages, and blame flooded everyone; certainly I felt alternately determined and terrified. The primary danger, perhaps tellingly, was that there could be no definitive control over random comments, things that might erupt in discussion, which no amount of planning could prevent. It is easy now to see that the conference's conflicts were at the heart of all the conflicts which boundary violations and their institutional management produce. Unregulated speech, the danger of knowledge, of feelings, of anguish, of rage. We were designing a conference as a kind of controlled manageable set of explosions perhaps and, as so frequently happens, the unconscious, collective and individual, took over.

Omnipotence and the analyst's melancholy: problems in self-care

A few years ago I finished an essay which was to be a chapter in a book on traumatic ruptures in clinical work (Deutsch, 2014). I was somewhat anxious about its topic as it detailed my return to work and analytic patients some months after the death of my husband. His death was sudden and very traumatic and I was concerned both about my capacities and the danger of misusing clinical situations either to hide or to be taken care of myself. In the paper,

I speculated on something that had certainly been on my mind. I was now, except for my gender, right in the demographic of analysts vulnerable to committing a boundary violation (Celenza, 1998). I was the right age, I was suffering a personal loss and its challenges. I had gone back to my analyst to discuss my circumstances. He was in the process of retiring and we talked about work both in situations of personal trauma and in the process of aging. Why did our profession begin to limit training analysts over 70? What was the thinking? 'Object hunger' he said, quietly. I held that perhaps old-fashioned term. It certainly packed a great emotional loading. All this was in my chapter. A close colleague read the paper and said quite clearly and definitively, about the issue of demographics and boundary violations, 'Take that out, doesn't belong there'. Without missing a beat, I said 'sure, ok' and removed the paragraph.

At the time, I was involved in the planning committee trying to organize the ultimately doomed conference on boundary violations. It was several weeks later, sitting in one of our committee meetings, listening to people talk about self-censorship and anxiety in relation to the entire issue, that I suddenly wondered—'What did I do?' Why did I whisk those thoughts and sentences away, scarcely registering what I was doing?

I put the paragraphs back in the essay and then I began to think about denial and—K and from there to the problem I had actually described: vulnerability. What is the relationship of boundary violations and some critical vulnerability in the analyst? There are certainly cases in which the analyst who does the boundary violation does so serially; there are problems that are characterological, not situational (Celenza & Hilsenroth, 1997).

But my essay and the enactments around it made me think about the barriers to talking about vulnerability and serious neglect of the analyst's self-care, very generally. This has been an issue I have been thinking and writing about for some time (Harris & Sinsheimer, 2008; Harris, 2009). At the heart of my concerns is a deep sense that self-care is often repudiated and even mocked by people in our field. Many analysts have in some part of their history a precocious demand to care for others. Healing can begin very early. Many of our most distinguished figures reveal or are revealed to have developed a vocation to heal and care for others, often at an early age. I have argued that this preoccupation, or early part of many of our formations, has both strengths and vulnerabilities. It can guide important adult and professional functions which anchor deep commitments to healing. But this early competence in caretaking depends on a defensive stance built on the actually shaky structures of omnipotence. Needs are banished. They are unnecessary, or shameful. Management of affect states and discomfort and longings are prized and rewarded. A bastion (Baranger & Baranger, 2008) is built, and often defended to the last breath.

This tendency to omnipotent functioning, responding to almost limitless demand, with heightened validation of suffering, creates a serious fault line in many analytic character structures, whether or not a boundary violation occurs. We are poor at self-care. Our most esteemed leaders, Ferenczi, Winnicott, Fairbairn, Fromm-Reichman, perhaps Freud as well, are rewarded and praised for extreme acts of care, acts perhaps often bordering on the masochistic.

A number of difficulties arise from this paucity of self-care and writing about self-care in our field. We don't seek help easily. We don't step towards a colleague who we fear needs help. The inevitably isolated aspects of therapeutic work deepen and can become hazardous. We have no collective mechanisms for help and support. If indeed, there are vulnerabilities because of loss and difficulties in personal life and relationships, the isolation of the analyst only deepens. To follow Bion on the need for two minds to allow one to think, it will often only be in some collective, group setting that thinking itself can be supported. These structures are sometimes on the books in institutes or work settings but rarely are they deployed for self-care or crises in self-care.

There are many reasons for this: capitalism, private practice as entrepreneurship … but habits of omnipotence also do their damage. I turn my attention now to a new model for justice and adjudicated conflicts but I do so also thinking that without the reform of habits of caretaking of ourselves and each other, collective efforts at finding resolutions will likely fail. There are plenty of personal issues and reasons that limit an individual's or a group's capacity to think and feel and dialogue. It will take enormous self-awareness and social will to expand these limits.

Restorative justice

Restorative justice (sometimes called reparative justice) is a model of crime and conflict resolution with roots in quite ancient cultural practices and in new models of jurisprudence (Gentile, 2015, 2018, this volume).

From the internet definition:

> Restorative Justice is a theory of justice that emphasizes repairing the harm caused by criminal behavior. It is best accomplished through cooperative processes that allow all willing stakeholders to meet, although other approaches are available when that is impossible. This can lead to transformation of people, relationships and communities.
>
> restorativejustice.org

The foundational principles of restorative justice have been summarized as follows:

1. Crime causes harm and justice should focus on repairing that harm.
2. The people most affected by the crime should be able to participate in its resolution.
3. The responsibility of the government is to maintain order and of the community to build peace.

If restorative justice were a building, it would have four cornerposts:

1. Inclusion of all parties
2. Encountering the other side
3. Making amends for the harm
4. Reintegration of the parties into their communities

To review: restorative justice …

- is a different way of thinking about crime and our response to crime
- focuses on repairing the harm caused by crime and reducing future harm through crime prevention

- ○ requires offenders to take responsibility for their actions and for the harm they have caused
- ○ seeks redress for victims, recompense by offenders and reintegration of both within the community
- ○ requires a cooperative effort by communities and the government

(Prison Fellowship International, 2017)

Looked at closely, this form of legal, community work seems perfectly suited for the problem of boundary violations in a psychoanalytic community. There is the understanding that many people at many levels have a stake in the process of identifying and sanctioning abuse. The model treats the community as a crucial ingredient in promoting change at any level. It also holds the promise or possibility of holding splits and alienation in less extreme forms.

Instead of expelling the criminal perpetrator from the community, the person remains in the community in a process with others. It is a process in which remorse, repair, and recovery would be worked on. This would involve the analyst, the patient and the community. This vision is of course idealized and hardly foolproof. In such a process within a psychoanalytic community, we would have to be highly motivated to think deeply about the problem, the problem of accountability, of community silence and to think psychoanalytically about these matters. Ironically, we might be one of the best trained groups to undertake this kind of thinking and group process but perhaps not well trained and prepared for the collective aspects of this task.

Looking at this model, one sees immediately how disastrous the current mechanisms for conflict resolution actually are. Our process is too often: exile, beheading, followed by silence. The problem is expelled, evacuated to a place of frozen otherness, all bad, all gone. In our current model, there is literally no way for a community to learn anything, to support members' education and development—even to understand what has happened or to speculate, perhaps, about why such a breakdown in ethical functioning has occurred. It seems that our usual individual and collective response mimics responses to trauma, freeze and dissociation, the very situations we work so hard with patients to unravel and relieve in their individual lives.

The question that has to be asked, however, is when and how would this be possible to enact? The brave and thoughtful holding that reparative justice offers is in marked contrast to the failed effort to have a conference in 2013. The problems seem to me to be not only legal and institutional, but fundamentally emotional. Legal sanctions, punishment, litigation may manage paranoia or vulnerability but they leave the institutions, groups and individuals still caught in lethal primitive states.

Yet, to me, one extremely important hope in a model of reparative justice (even just to have this discussed) is the possibility of avoiding beheadings and the execution of demons. If we can keep the danger and hatred inside the system, we might have a chance to understand it.

References

Aron, L. (1995). The internalized primal scene. *Psychoanalytic Dialogues* 5(2): 195–237.

Aron, L. (2000). Self-Reflexivity and the Therapeutic Action of Psychoanalysis. *Psychoanalytic Psychology*, 17(4): 667–689.

Baranger, W. & Baranger, M. (2008). The psychoanalytic situation as a dynamic field. *International Journal of Psychoanalysis* 89: 795–826.

Bion, W.R. (1962). *Learning from experience.* London: Tavistock.

Bion, W.R. (1970). *Attention and interpretation.* London: Tavistock.

Celenza, A. (1998). Precursors to therapist sexual misconduct: Preliminary findings. *Psychoanalytic Psychology* 15: 378–397.

Celenza, A. (2007). *Sexual boundary violations: Therapeutic, supervisory, and academic contexts.* New York: Jason Aronson.

Celenza, A. & Hilsenroth, M. (1997). Personality characteristics of mental health professionals who have engaged in sexualized dual relationships: A Rorschach investigation. *Bulletin of the Menninger Clinic* 61: 90–107.

Davies, J.M. (1996). Linking the 'pre-analytic' with the post-classical: Integration, dissociation, and the multiplicity of unconscious processes. *Contemporary Psychoanalysis* 32: 553–576.

Davis, T. (2021). Rehabilitation in a boundary violation from the perspective of the transgressor. *This volume* (pp. 45–59).

Deutsch, R. (Ed.). (2014). *Traumatic ruptures: Abandonment and betrayal in the analytic relationship.* New York and London: Routledge.

Dimen, M. (2011). Lapsus linguae, or a slip of the tongue: A sexual violation in an analytic treatment and its personal and theoretical aftermath. *Contemporary Psychoanalysis* 47(1): 35–79.

Dimen, M. (2017). Eight topics: A conversation on sexual boundary violations between Charles Amrhein and Muriel Dimen. *Psychoanalytic Psychology* 34(2): 169–174.

Gabbard, G.O. & Lester, E.P. (1995). *Boundaries and boundary violations in psychoanalysis.* NY: Basic Books.

Gabbard, G.O. & Peltz, M.L. (2001). Speaking the unspeakable: Institutional reactions to boundary violations by training analysts. *Journal of the American Psychoanalytic Asssociation* 49: 659–673.

Gentile, K. (2015). Personal communication.

Gentile, K. (2018). When the cat guards the canary: Using bystander intervention towards community-based response. *This volume* (pp. 77–99).

Goldberg, P. (2008), Cataastrophic change, communal dreaming and the counter-catastropic personality. Paper read at the 4th Annual EBOR Conference, Seattle, WA. November 1, 2008.

Harris, A. (2009). You must remember this. *Psychoanalytic Dialogues* 19(1): 2–21.

Harris, A. & Sinsheimer, K. (2008). The analyst's vulnerability: Preserving and fine-tuning analytic bodies. In F. Anderson (Ed.), *Bodies in treatment.* New York: Routledge.

Jurist, E., Alpert, J.L., & Steinberg, A.L. (Eds.). (2017). Special issue: Sexual boundary violations. *Psychoanalytic Psychology* 34(2).

Katz, G. (2014). *The play within the play: The enacted dimension of psychoanalytic process.* New York, NY: Routledge.

Pinsky, E. (2011). The Olympian delusion. *Journal of the American Psychoanalytic Association* 59: 351–375.

Prison Fellowship International (2017). https://pfi.org

Slochower, J. (2017, this volume). Don't tell anyone. *Psyhoanalytic Psychology* 34(2): 195–200.

Stein, R. (2005). Why perversion?: 'False love' and the perverse pact. *International Journal of Psychoanalysis* 86(3): 775–799.

Winnicott, D.W. (1949). Hate in the countertransference. *International Journal of Psychoanalysis* 30: 69–74.

Chapter 5

When the cat guards the canary

Using bystander intervention towards community-based response

Katie Gentile

As we know, when the analytic couple is stuck in a clinical impasse, the emergence of a "third" position can create the space necessary for reflection and meaning making (Benjamin, 2004), enabling the dyad to come to a new way of being. Without this space for reflection the dyad can easily get trapped in a rigid, temporally linear repetition. In this chapter, I propose that the field of psychoanalysis itself is stuck in a similar kind of impasse, in which we seem unable to develop a creative response to the serial crisis of major boundary violations even in the upper ranks of our professional organizations. Like any stuck dyad, or shamed family, the field of psychoanalysis has, for the most part, chosen repetition and the practice of relying on psychoanalysts to "police" our own, keeping the family secret. Like a cat guarding the canary, this practice not only puts our patients (not to mention analysts who are at risk, and the profession itself) in jeopardy; it repeats the very structure of a familial act of disavowal, which, as recent research has shown, tends to produce transgenerational patterns of trauma (e.g. Faimberg, 2005, etc. Levin, 2014). This chapter uses the example of recent strategies developed in the college setting as a way of suggesting, from a perspective outside the field, how psychoanalysis might create for itself a more viable ethical third. Indeed, the experience of boundary violations in higher education, whose resemblance to psychoanalysis is often downplayed in the psychoanalytic profession, provides an interesting opportunity for experiments in thinking about our ethical practices and for generating new and more effective ways of defining and engaging the issues of prevention, threat and violation.

Introduction – disavowed multiplicities and "family/ies" secrets

In 2011, the United States Department of Education filed charges against Yale University for its failure to provide women students with equal access to education. The suit was the culmination of years of complaints from women students who endured what was described as a culture of verbal and physical violence against women. The students used Title IX to support their claim that the university's refusal to address or investigate reports of sexual harassment, stalking, rape and attempted rape on campus was not merely the toleration of, but the creation of a hostile environment for women students, limiting their access to education.[1]

In this chapter I am taking the tack of using an external example in order to better identify and understand similar issues in the psychoanalytic space. My example is that of college-based systems of intervention to address, investigate and prevent sexual violence. In doing this, I want to present a specific model of intervention based on the idea of breaking the vicious cycle that perpetuates victim-perpetrator dynamic, which can silence and paralyze the potential response of communities to problems in their midst. I am not attempting to make a direct comparison between sexual boundary violations in the psychoanalytic setting with the various kinds of boundary trouble that occur within the college setting; rather, I wish to explore the responses to these problems that have been generated within the college communities. I believe that psychoanalysts stand to learn from the practices that have been developing in the university setting and to learn about what has been considered effective in these contexts. My approach is based on the fundamentally psychoanalytic idea that transference-countertransference or "field" dynamics can become self-enclosing without the benefit of a third position from which the space for reflection can emerge (Dimen, 2011). This chapter is one attempt at creating an outside position from which we might be able to compare, contrast, and look inside psychoanalysis anew.

There are vast differences between a college community and the psychoanalytic setting; most obviously, the latter holds privacy and confidentiality as central to its process. For the psychoanalytic process, transference and countertransference are fuel to the work that needs to be done. According to Baranger and Baranger (2008) the contract or "promise" of therapy is that the therapist will provide "help in resolving conflicts through interpretations and promises confidentiality and abstantion from any intervention in the other's 'real' life" (p. 796). This promise determines behavior so that analytic interactions maintain an "as if" quality, which they compare to seeing a play. As they note, an analyst should be able to differentiate the actor playing Hamlet from Hamlet, or in this paper, the patient playing a seducer from a seducer. The analytic situation, then, is akin to a dream to be held and examined but not acted out.

But erotic dreams and transferences have been conceptualized as being oftentimes outside of our control. Elise describes erotic transference like a rip tide (Elise, 2015). This analogy differs with that of the slippery slope in a number of important ways. According to Elise, the slippery slope conjures a clear visual gradation that implies with "careful footing, where one does not stray" from the clear non-slope path, one can avoid slipping. In fact, as she observes, there is no clear path to avoid the slope altogether.

Anyone who has had the pleasure of swimming in an ocean knows the danger of rip tides and the ways they are often invisible to the untrained eye. The rip tide only becomes apparent once you are caught in it, being pushed and pulled out to sea. It is a visceral analogy, felt in the muscles of your body that feel the stretch and strain. Even the best and strongest swimmers are no match for a riptide. No indeed. That's why at most beaches now there is a drawing of exactly how to swim out of a riptide. Only by swimming *in* the riptide, not against it, will one make their way out of the pull. One is to observe the tide: not to fight it by swimming away, or through it in an attempt to get to shore; but to maintain a focus on the shoreline, feeling the pull of the tide, but swimming parallel as long as needed until the tide recedes and one is freed to swim back to shore. In other words, respecting the force of affects while exploring them, always keeping a firm eye on the shore – the "as if" quality of the analytic space – is *the* work of psychoanalysis. One may be able to predict the conditions for a rip tide, but not the exact location and force of one, how it will tug at the body and destabilize. One can imagine in advance what to do – train oneself to swim out of it, use knowledge and theory as a "lifejacket" (Elise, personal communication) – but doing so in the moment is a frightening challenge. We can learn theories about erotic transference and read papers from clinicians who have a facility for acknowledging and working with it, but each tide will present unique and frightening challenges. Furthermore, it is just these theories of psychoanalysis and the frame, Elise's "life-jackets," that are often disavowed, thrown out, or manipulated to justify boundary violations. These acts reinforce what Honig and Barron (2013), Foehl (2005), and Levine (2010b) have observed, that analytic boundary violations damage the psychoanalytic community and profession at large, and are aggressive acts against the profession. Additionally, the felt experience of these violations is one of multi-layered institutional betrayal. Initially theorized by Smith and Freyd (2014), institutional betrayal is a central component of trauma for most survivors of sexual misconduct, describing the affective investment in an ideological apparatus like "school" or "the justice system" (Doyle, 2015, p. 35), and how betrayal by these institutional bodies result in multiple levels of traumatic response (Gentile, in review). Thus, these boundary violations need to be conceptualized and understood to be community-based transgressions demanding a community-based, institution level response.

Professors and colleges do not have the same responsibility for holding a relational process, including understanding the multiplicities of self-experiences and conscious and unconscious motivations and intentionalities (Bromberg, 1998; Mitchell, 2000). Psychoanalysts are supposed to understand that these multiplicities in addition to the concept of mutuality (see Aron, 1996) mean we never really know how our colleagues interact with patients because each relational encounter is an opportunity to come into being anew. Thus, we really do not know what happens behind any closed door. Yet these theories do not seem to help us comprehend when someone we know transgresses. We find ourselves caught like the neighbor of a perpetrator who on the local news can only repeat "but they were such a nice person, prolific writer, wonderful mentor ...." or as Foehl (2005) wrote, "how could this happen to me?"

Yet despite structural differences, as social bodies, psychoanalysis and the academy have both chosen a similar tactic to deal with violations: policing, investigating, and disciplining their own. Indeed, this is the same biased and inadequate, closed system used by the Catholic Church in investigating child sexual abuse, the U.S. military to investigate and prosecute sexual assaults (one of the lead prosecutors was recently arrested for sexual assault himself), and many U.S. police departments – organizations that have received criticisms from many psychoanalytic groups for their biased and victim-blaming investigative procedures. Yet, historically, boundary violations within psychoanalysis have been dealt with (if they were dealt with) by peers and/or internal institutional and professional ethics committees. Police are not called to investigate; after all, sex between an adult patient and her/his analyst is not a crime. Perhaps a state ethics board is notified – *perhaps*. But the protection of the institute's reputation and the identity of the accused take precedence. After all, one accusation can cause violent ripples throughout a training setting and could potentially ruin one's livelihood (see Wallace, 2007; Ruskin, 2011) for detailed accounts of the impact of accusations and investigations of boundary violations in institute settings). Here the traditional form of victim-blaming in cases of sexual violence is institutionalized, as the main protections often go to the accused. The accuser, by mentioning the accusation, can be sued for defamation. Indeed Blechner (2014) refers to Celenza's (2007) research indicating that psychoanalysts who do sue the accusing patient receive more favorable responses from ethics boards than those who do not respond aggressively. Despite these informal protections for the accused, both universities and analytic communities have recently been exposed to high profile lawsuits.

Discussion of sexual boundary violations cannot help but be shaped and limited by the familiar doer/done to, Judeo-Christian based, judicial structure (Butler, 1997; Benjamin, 2004; Cornell, 2010) for participants. Not only is there limited grey area in that binary, there is also limited capacity to imagine one side without the other. Psychoanalytic notions of enactment and trauma have helped us better understand how these positions may shift and how the abuser can become the abused and vice versa (Davies & Frawley, 1992). But in these theories the binary oppositions remain firm even as participants themselves change roles. Using examples from a college/university setting I am hoping to create some space outside this judicial binary, where accountability and shame can be held, fostered and reflected upon.

Postcolonial theorists (Spivak, 1988; Mohanty, 2004), philosophers and legal scholars (Tronto, 1994; Oliver, 2001; Cornell, 2010) describe witnessing and testimony that include perpetrator accountability as integral to the creation of a third space of resolution, healing, or what psychoanalysts would also identify as moving out of enactment. Shame, here, is not to be avoided like a hot potato. Of course the act of avoidance and the shame itself can close down psychic space for reflection, but we are ruled by our own narcissism when we insist it can only do that. We grant it tremendous power. Shaming, as Mary Douglas (1966) observed years ago, is one of the most important and effective tools of social organizations. To avoid shame is to shield perpetrators from the effects and impact of their actions, which denies them of their dignity. It denies the pain and dignity of the victims, including the pain of the community. After all, there is no space to make amends without shame. Accountability then requires that the perpetrator hold shame; it is a necessary component of recognition for both victims and the community as a whole. Philosopher Kelly Oliver (2001, 2004), referencing postcolonial and critical race theorists, describes how the "other" functions to hold and embody the shameful affects for the colonizers. Thus, creating the capacities to shift shame back to the transgressor, who shares it with the potentially enabling community body, is key. They must be supported to hold their own shame, to examine it, to move through it (Gentile, 2017a). This will be elaborated upon later in the chapter.

Certainly sexual relations, whether in the context of teaching/ mentoring students or within psychoanalytic settings, always touch on questions of consent. Consent is so important we have even created an additional level for research and clinical work, called "informed" consent. Legally, consent can only operate between positions of equal cognitive capacity and implies a subject with only conscious and non-contradictory motivations and intentions. Animals, children, adults with developmental disabilities and adults under the influence of drugs or alcohol cannot legally consent to sexual activities as it is assumed these subjects cannot exercise the necessary judgment to understand the situation to which they are consenting. In this legal ideal, there is no room for the temporal evolutions of desire (Saketopoulou, 2010) and self-experiencing (Gentile, 2013a, 2015) that render motivation and intention assemblaged potentialities that are always context dependent. Additionally, if we are serious about regression, then technically, at best, patients can only exercise consent initially, when the frame of the analytic treatment is being negotiated. Once the treatment is in progress, consent to any changes in the relationship could be considered impossible, and certainly be seen as a function of transference or/ and countertransference. (This is not to say these forces are not operating immediately upon the first phone contact or websearch). Of course, this position is directly opposite that taken by Harry Smith, who defended himself against accusations of sexual boundary violations with a patient by saying that because the patient was a psychologist herself, she understood the power of transference and countertransference and thus exercised consent to a sexual relationship (Herman, 2012). In order to be a political person capable of consent one needs protected areas of fantasy, desire, and public imagination (Cornell, in Skerrett, 2010). A psychoanalytic dyad might be a means to the development of the capacity for consent, but by definition, the relationship is not based on equal capacities in the moment. One consistent issue with describing patients being unable to exercise consent is that it can be seen as patronizing and disempowering. In our neoliberal world that clings to the fetish of self-regulation, balance, and unfettered individualistic agency (Layton, 2010; Gentile, 2013a), to question consent is to undermine coherent and legible subjectivity and value. But we are not individual subjects, as relational psychoanalysis in particular knows (Aron, 1996; Bromberg, 1998; Mitchell, 2000). Moreover, the psychoanalytic relationship is one formed by dynamics of power that are carefully articulated by "the frame." Even in the most relational approach, analyst and patient may be collaborating and we may theorize about relationally emergent subjectivities; but it is the analyst who after 45 minutes ends the interaction and collects the payment from the assemblage who is identified as being the patient.

Blechner (2014 refers to Mackler (2006) with the observation that it is the patient's role to try to seduce the therapist and the therapist's role to analyze that. If the analyst goes along with the transference and allows the seduction to materialize into action, then it is the therapist who has seduced the patient, however disguised or overt the seduction was. Thus consent in the context of psychoanalysis is not theoretically possible.

Boundary violations reach beyond consent because by violating, the professional fails to hold up their end of the bargain. They act aggressively to destroy the process of treatment. This is not something to which a patient can consent.

Sexual violence in the college context

Returning to the academy, research indicates that dating and sexual violence is common among college students, with prevalence rates from 14% (Dekeseredy & Kelly, 1993) to about 40% (White & Koss, 1991). A blended method study of dating violence, sexual assault and stalking indicated that local commuter students at an urban campus had violence rates of 36%, higher than the national average (Gentile et al., 2007). Although very common, until recently most colleges considered such violence a problem best addressed by women's centers and similar student services. The fact that most of these entities are usually underfunded and understaffed, with limited capacities to address violence on campuses, has not been considered relevant. But when the university/college's response to sexual violence is approached as a Title IX funding issue (this has happened due to pressure from student groups), suddenly there is a need to develop an institutionalized systematic response.

I was the director of a college women's center for over 10 years. The position was part clinical, part programming for students and the community, and part faculty – research and teaching. Like most college women's centers, I dealt with countless cases of intimate partner violence, rape and sexual assault between students as well as cases of students who had sex with staff members or professors. The women's center, like many such centers within college campuses, gradually became responsible for the development and implementation of violence prevention programs around issues of sexual and intimate partner violence and harassment. Prevention and intervention was considered part of complying with The Clery Act. This act was signed into law in 1990, as a response to the rape and murder of a freshman student, Jeanne Clery in 1986. Her campus knew it had a problem with a serial rapist but it had not reported this fact to parents or students. The Clery Act mandates open reporting of crimes on campuses for schools receiving federal funding. The Act does not address prevention or intervention directly.

It is important to understand the ramifications of locating prevention within women's centers. First, as research demonstrates, most women's centers are significantly underfunded, most receiving no operational funds from colleges (Kasper, 2004). Most women's centers have limited staff and space to undertake a school-wide prevention effort. Lastly, many women's centers are not highly respected on campus either because of their identified mission (i.e. women's empowerment, activism and feminism) or/and because of the traditional Cartesian split between body and mind: student activities are considered the touchy feely body, split off as separate, unrelated to the intellectual academic mission of the college. Thus, situating prevention within women's centers can send a message to the campus that this effort is not considered to be important.

Around 2009, after years of agitation by women's center directors, a university wide activist student group started making noise about the lack of uniformity in the treatment and policies for sexual-based violence on campuses. My college is one of 19 campuses throughout New York City. The main University administration wields its power selectively, deciding what issues it can mandate. A policy addressing sexual violence, we were told, was not an area they felt they could mandate for individual campuses. But the students were riding a cultural wave where prevention was seen as extremely important. The Virginia Tech shooter had a file in various offices that included a history of stalking behaviors. There was a nationwide push for the development of prevention specialist task forces on campuses.[2] Women students were beginning to use Title IX to sue schools for failing to provide access to education. So the University listened and created a committee to establish a university-wide policy.

The shift in the use of Title IX cannot be underestimated.[3] Although it was initiated as a response to violence, Title IX has been described most often in relation to access to athletics. Yet, under Title IX, schools have a great deal of responsibility to act in the face of accusations, not just proven incidents, of rape, sexual assault or harassment and intimate partner violence. Additionally colleges were supposed to follow the "knew or should have known" standard of intervention (Murphy, personal communication). This makes colleges responsible for violence based on the atmosphere and conditions of the campus. Given the usually private nature of rape, sexual assault and harassment and intimate partner violence, this means schools have a responsibility to act even if there is not clear evidence to prosecute. Does one have guaranteed access to education if one is raped on campus, or seduced by a professor, or if one is able to successfully seduce one's professor? (Does one have adequate access to a clinical relationship if one is able to seduce one's analyst or be seduced by their analyst?) Title IX was used in the courts as the women claimed the school's refusal to investigate or/and discipline perpetrators not only reinforced violent behaviors but constituted discrimination that hindered the women students' participation in their education. Using Title IX in this way also shifted the discourse of college prevention work, focussing on the realities that the very atmosphere of many college campuses hindered women students' participation in their education. The college/ university had a responsibility to create an *atmosphere* where such violence was unacceptable. There would need to be clear definitions of what constituted the various forms of violence. All the details of this would have to be thought through and addressed: ramifications for perpetrators, adequate support and advocacy for victims, accountability for students and the college at large, and the development and implementation of prevention-based curriculum for all incoming students.

This approach also necessitated an epistemological shift. The microaggressions and macroaggressions (Sue et al., 2007), including sexual and intimate partner violence, were recast not as private issues between students but as significant problems that the university/college had a legal (and ethical) responsibility not just to address, but to prevent. This approach is challenging not least because it disrupts Western culture's comfortable split between public and private spaces. Here colleges would have to find ways to influence the private spaces of interpersonal interactions and actively prevent certain behaviors occurring in those spaces.

This tide of prevention and intervention was only heightened by the media attention on Yale University that was facing huge fines based on Title IX. Public and private universities that rely on federal funding for student loans or/and operational costs were forced to take notice. So I became part of a committee tasked with developing a policy to address intimate partner violence, stalking and sexual assault.

The outline of the policy we wrote involved the creation of definitions, ways sexual violence could be identified, campus points of entry for students, how cases would be investigated, and disciplinary steps that could be taken. This might seem cut and dried, but consider the seemingly simple part of identifying entry points. We knew from experience that affected students sought out the assistance of professors, counselors, coaches, mentors in student activities, women's centers, security personnel and their student peers. This meant that all these constituents needed to be trained how to identify cases of sexual violence and to intervene at their respective levels of responsibility (i.e. a counselor would intervene differently from a security officer). Additionally, the training curriculum needed to address potential biases about different forms of sexual violence (including trainees' potential tendencies toward victim-blaming, downplaying certain forms of violence, and ignoring harassment, including homophobic and misogynous hate speech), while communicating an established protocol for reporting sexual violence. In practice, this gets very complicated. Where should reports go? To the Dean of Students? To Security? Both? But when cases began in the Counseling Center, confidentiality trumped any reporting protocol. And who would develop the training curriculum? Who would conduct the various trainings? How could the policy committee convince college Presidents that directors needed to attend trainings and that directors needed to prioritize staff trainings when the Presidents themselves might not see the urgency? As I learned, my college enjoyed strong top-down support for the work of the policy, but not every campus was so fortunate.

That was just training. What about the team identified for investigation? Title IX and the Clery Act make it clear that campus police cannot be the only investigators for crimes and victims must be urged to contact local police on their own.

Nationally many universities and colleges had pressured students not to call local police. They kept investigations internal, allowing them to pad statistics. Universities and colleges sometimes took months or years to investigate accusations, leaving the accuser in a potentially dangerous physical and psychological limbo. For instance, does a student continue to go to a class where a professor is accused of harassment, risking a failing grade if they do not? What about the student who fears returning to campus for fear of running into a perpetrator? Investigations must occur in a "timely manner" but what does this mean? What about students whose campus jobs are at risk if they have to avoid specific areas in order to comply with restraining orders? What about students who are accused? What are their rights to educational access? How can they be denied access to the campus or to their classes or extracurricular activities during the investigation? Indeed, like the analyst, students too can sue for discrimination when accused. These are real life examples that only hint at the complications involved in seemingly simple steps.

Disrupting binary dynamics of victim–perpetrator

In the end, what made the university policy particularly progressive was its focus on bystander intervention. Bystander intervention is based on the idea that people act depending on the behaviors of those around them. As social psychologists know, the more witnesses there are, the less likely it is that individuals will respond. Bystander intervention focuses on examining some of the reasons people choose not to respond in certain situations. This approach disrupts socially reinforced habits of victim-blaming, thereby helping to shift social norms. It also shifts responsibility to both men and women, but does so with an understanding of differential positions of cultural power. In other words, yes, women have a strong substantial role, but unfortunately within a patriarchal system most men are more influenced by the opinions and behaviors of other men. It follows that male bystanders have an important role to play. Bystander intervention begins from the premise that most people are not violent, yet stay silent when faced with violence because they lack the confidence or knowledge to intervene. Bystander intervention is based on the ontological assumption that people want to intervene or find a way to stop the violence.

Organized around bystander intervention, our prevention materials and curriculum for faculty, staff and students was focussed not on the gendered binary of doer-done to, victim–perpetrator, but on the third party, the bystander. Research on prevention efforts in colleges has found that one-shot programs are not effective and in some cases can result in increased misogynous and homophobic violence (Morrison et al., 2004). Based on my experience of organizing large-scale, campus-wide prevention programs though, one shot may be all one gets if one is lucky. Usually you get a flier buried in a packet of pages and pages of orientation information that is most likely thrown away by the student. But if prevention focusses on engaging students as bystanders, they are more likely to listen and less likely to respond with a backlash. Here the rigid oppositional victim and perpetrator positions fade to the background and the bystander, the witness, is elevated and made agentic. The focus of trainings is on helping students identify sexual violence, not by positioning them as potential victims or perpetrators but as bystanders. Students are asked to recall situations where they saw violence occurring. They are asked to identify the violence. Then they are asked to describe how they felt as witnesses to the violence. Most recall intense and shameful feelings of vulnerability, helplessness and powerlessness and they are able to identify and describe these most often because they were not the direct victim or perpetrator. Some recall considering or indeed enacting violent physical or verbal responses. Then scenarios are presented from these real life stories and students are walked through ways they might intervene (if safe), or alert an authority; how they might talk to a friend who was assaulted or harassed; and most importantly, how they can talk to a friend who crossed the line themselves. Having organized and implemented these trainings, I have found students respond quite positively to being coached to help victims. But when I open up the idea of intervening with a perpetrator the discussion initially falls silent. Eyes drop to the floor, bodies shift, twitch or freeze. Then one by one, students open up about experiences they have already had with friends who perpetrated some physically or verbally violent act where they did not know what to do. Not surprisingly, students described wanting to disavow and avoid any future feelings of powerlessness and helpless vulnerability, meaning they employed strategies that allowed them to avoid acknowledging future micro/macro aggressions and/or supported their own use of such aggression in their own interactions. Providing tools for intervening, even if the tool was just an active reflection of that powerlessness, results in a disruption of the victim–perpetrator dynamic. It creates the space for a third position that is not completely devoid of the others, but at the very least, has more space for reflection and movement.

Bystander intervention does not just shift individual student behaviors; it creates a shift in the campus culture. It is a system that cannot fail to help change the campus atmosphere and the cultural body. It creates a way to gradually disassemble the dissociative tendency to project badness elsewhere, where it usually comes to settle on persons or groups who stand for the *other*. The bystander may be the third, the witness, but it is clear that bystander position comes with close proximity to both the victim and perpetrator. Here the knowledge that we could all be victim or perpetrator is held and used to fuel not dissociation but reflective and realistic action to become an agentic bystander.

Accountability within this model is shared with the bystander, who has a responsibility to intervene in some way. The pressures on the victim–perpetrator dyad are diffused as the bystander, and thus the community body, shares the shame and accountability.

A psychoanalytic bystander

Clearly college settings differ from psychoanalytic spaces in a number of ways, but perhaps institutes can take note of what the academy has found helpful and most effective (understanding that efficacy in this area is complex and difficult to measure). Not surprisingly given theories of the repetition of violence and trauma, situating prevention and intervention within a community can be effective. This requires supporting all community members in their capacities to be agentic and powerful bystanders, which relies on clearly articulated procedures for reporting (including transparent ramifications and consequences of reporting), transparent protocols for intervention and accountability that is consistent and apparent to the community, including maintaining a clear channel of communication throughout the "timely" investigation. These procedures need to be communicated to non-candidate patients as well. Keeping the community in the dark or being inconsistent collapses the bystander agency, pulling the community back into the rigid position of victim/perpetrator and functions to create more anxiety and dissociation (Wallace, 2007). Thus, community building is a powerful form of accountability and functions toward the collective containment and processing of shame. Again, shame that is actively held is able to be metabolized by the community and the perpetrator and more likely to be able to be used toward transformation and not paralysis of a collapse of reflection (Gentile, 2017a; in review).

These ideals of bystander agency are just ideals if there is not community accountability. This accountability, as described in the college setting, requires the capacity to create and sustain an atmosphere that does not tolerate abuse in any form. But maintaining this cultural atmosphere requires engaging in a continual on-going process as groups, like individuals, will typically retreat to positions and interactions that are familiar, even when they are the positions of oppression and violence (Bion, 1961/1989). So for instance as I was finishing this chapter I was asked to join a meeting at my university because some administrators were planning to re-interpret an important part of the policy that would guarantee less support for victims, thus, fewer victims would report. Had the lawyer I worked with on writing the policy not reached out to me to join her, the policy would have been re-interpreted based on the structural preferences of the administration and not the continuing progression of community building and changing the campus atmosphere. Community accountability is an ongoing process that requires a great deal of vigilance.

The bullying of candidates, younger community members, and those with less professional prestige described by Levin (2014), is also an obvious deterrent to this form of community building. So too is the perhaps more common "cult of personality" that develops in institutes, a dynamic that favors those members with professional prestige, granting them positions of power, authority, and decision-making. The dynamics of this cult of personality can position certain members above the law. This hierarchical arrangement is quite dangerous. How does a candidate approach, intercede with, and question the behaviors, actions, words of an established or even famous analyst/teacher/supervisor? How does a colleague with less power question the actions or behaviors of a more famous one without feeling a threat to professional growth, such as threats to future opportunities to teach, publish, and present, and/or to receive patient referrals? To be effective, speaking up cannot come with professional or personal punishment. Thus, all members of the community not only have to be aware of the procedures of speaking up and reporting. These procedures need to be implemented by a committee of people at varying levels of professional development and prestige, including candidates. There also needs to be strict, clear, adhered to guidelines for disciplining attempts at retribution. Many cases I have worked on were turned to the victim's favor when the perpetrator or community members began harassing the person who reported. Retribution is often the most provable, yet most ignored, violation.

A community-based response, though, also requires intervention for the perpetrator or professional at risk of violation. As mentioned previously, colleges have to have a multi-department committee that takes reports from the community, works to identify the students and faculty at risk, and helps determine appropriate interventions. Institutes could have similar committee-based intervention teams. Such a committee could be used to help those in fear of violating. However, due to the confidential and private nature of psychoanalytic work, the most important form of intervention is interpersonal, helping members operationalize risky behaviors, identify them in themselves and others, and learn appropriate forms of intervening for the psychoanalytic setting. However, psychoanalysis gets in deep trouble when it uses the confidential nature of the work as an excuse for special rules, codes of ethics, and/or processes of investigation and reporting. It may be a unique setting but the operations of power, privilege, and abuse are universal.

Additionally, as colleges have found, procedures need to be in place to accept and investigate anonymous reporting. This is a step my university was unwilling to take, but campuses with anonymous reporting tend to cultivate an atmosphere much less tolerant of violence. (It is important to note that many campuses, including mine, refused this form of reporting supposedly not out of fear of receiving too many unfounded accusations but out of a concern for being able to provide support for the reporting victim). Thus institutes and communities need to develop channels for anonymous reporting that are formal enough to be differentiated from gossip, but still accessible for those fearing retribution or those who see reporting as a form of professional suicide, which, unfortunately, it can be.

At this point one may be associating to other forms of witnessing and community intervention, such as the Truth and Reconciliation Committees, where bystanders – i.e. other community members, were made agentic witnesses, active members of an institutionalized system of accountability, or one might recall the origins of witnessing in women of color's ideas of testimony functioning to (re)unite the cultural, political and personal/psychology (Beverley, 1992; Smith & Watson, 1992. Although bystander intervention is similar to these ideas of witnessing, it goes beyond ideas of witnessing written about in psychoanalysis.

First off, recent psychoanalytic translations of witnessing do not always make links to the cultural and political nor do they explore their impact on subjectivities (Gentile, 2013b, 2017b). Certainly psychoanalytic ideas of witnessing have been linked to the creation of a similar third space, a "live" or "moral third" (Feldmen & Laub, 1992; Benjamin, 2009; Gerson, 2009; Boulanger, 2012) and can provide a way of entering another's subjectivity, a deep form of recognition and perspective (Benjamin, 2004, 2009). The bystander does enter into both the victim's and perpetrator's respective subjectivities, attempting to engage both if only in thought.

One could see bystander intervention as being close to Ullman's (2006) use of Margalit's (2002) idea of moral witnessing, where the witness reports on and documents "a reality of human suffering inflicted by evil policies" (p. 183). Analysts writing about witnessing often use the term "evil," locating it squarely in the "other," a third party, not-me, not-you, but "them" (Poland, 2000: Grand, 2002, 2003; Boulanger, 2012). As observed elsewhere (Gentile, 2013b), this can function to triangulate, pulling the patient close through a presumed identification of goodness and distance from evil, such that we-together are not-them, not bad. Bystander intervention demands evil and goodness be held together within the bystander. In psychoanalytic witnessing the violence is conceptualized as having happened outside the dyad (albeit potentially being re-enacted within it). The culpability of the analyst for current and historical violence is typically missing in most accounts (see Gentile,

2013b). For the bystander this ethical relating has to be earned through the process of intervening and actively challenging the violation. Only by speaking up is the bystander differentiated from the perpetrator or victim. Thus, the bystander is motivated by "an obligation ... to respond in a way that opens up rather than closes off the possibility of response by others" (Oliver, 2001, p. 201), an obligation to restore dignity (Ullman, 2006) to one's self as well as to the victim and perpetrator. This response-ability and restoration of dignity requires holding people and institutional bodies accountable for what may be shame-full actions.

In some ways this ideal of bystander intervention is also in line with restorative justice, where the victim and perpetrator mediate not what happened but how to materialize accountability and reparations in an attempt to restore justice to both the victim and the community (see Daly, 2006; Koss et al., 2014; Gentile, 2017a). As I have written else-where (Gentile, 2017a), The unique value of restorative justice is that it does not dissociate the perpetrator, splitting them off from the community. Instead they are held within the communal body where they are expected to enact a caring and responsible accountability, usually out-lined by the victim and the community. As I have written elsewhere (Gentile, 2017a), such a model would disrupt the typical dissociative tendencies where the perpetrator is identified as the container of all the misconduct and split off from the community that then remains sup-posedly evacuated of all wrongdoing. However, as Daly (2006) observes with adolescent participants in restorative justice, this tech-nique requires that the perpetrator be accountable for their actions. This can be a tall order not just with adolescents but with sexual boundary violators who insist they have done nothing wrong. Further, restorative justice relies on the fantasies that justice can be restored and that there was a former time of justice. In a culture that often relies on victim blaming in cases of sexual misconduct and boundary violations, restoration is to a future, not a past of justice.

As I have written throughout this chapter, the academic setting is different from the clinical setting but perhaps some links can be made to psychoanalytic institutes and other psychoanalytic communities. Perhaps some basic ideas of bystander intervention, namely the emphasis on community building, the roles of community members to act and respond and in turn create conditions for responding, can help shape institutional approaches to dealing with sexual boundary violations. Here ethics training would entail creating the conditions for responding – response-ability. Violations would be seen not only as the destructive actions of an individual, but an indication of the shame-full and destructive atmosphere created and sustained by the institute and community. Imagine a training institute, a psychoanalytic community, actively promoting an atmosphere where analysts, patients, supervisors, candidates, and faculty had mutual accountability, mutual response-ability and mutual investment in the process of a just psycho-analysis.

Notes

1 As this chapter went to press, the new Secretary of Education, Betsy DeVos, made it clear she would not continue to enforce Title IX investigations.
2 These teams are known as BIT – Behavioral Intervention Teams. The national guidelines recommend members be representatives from academic affairs, students' services – including counselors and liaisons with women's centers – security personnel, and legal council. BIT teams meet regularly to discuss any students who have been identified as being disruptive or potentially at risk for failing academically. It is a prevention-based model of intervention.
3 After this chapter was written, the United States Department of Education's Office for Civil Rights created a Dear Colleague Letter for all college campuses. It outlined strict guidelines for addressing sexual misconduct on campuses. Some feel this letter gives colleges more latitude to dodge responsibility to respond to reports of violence, as it fails to outline what is a timely investigation. Indeed some universities have concluded investigations years after the report, when the offender was about to graduate, thereby avoiding need for punishment or dismissal. Soon after this letter, the U.S. press finally began covering the slew of sexual assault allegations on college campuses and the often poor procedures for investigating and supporting victims and holding perpetrators accountable. Related to this coverage was the continuing failure of colleges to place sexual assaults within a cultural and campus atmosphere that condones male violence against women and other forms of gender-based violence. Unfortunately this DCL approached sexual misconduct from a criminal justice stance, with less emphasis on community accountability (Gentile, 2017).

References

Aron, L. (1996). *A meeting of minds: Mutuality in psychoanalysis*. Hillsdale, NJ: The Analytic Press.

Baranger, M. & Baranger, W. (2008). The analytic situation as a dynamic field. *International Journal of Psychoanalysis*, *89*: 795–826.

Benjamin, J. (2004). Beyond doer and done to: An intersubjective view of thirdness. *Psychoanalytic Quarterly*, *LXXIII*(1): 5–46.

Benjamin, J. (2009). A relational psychoanalysis perspective on the necessity of acknowledging failure in order to restore the facilitating and containing features of the intersubjective relationship (the shared third). *International Journal of Psychoanalysis*, *90*: 441–450.

Beverley, J. (1992). The margin at the center: On *Testimonio* (Testimonial narrative). In S. Smith & J. Watson (Eds.), *De/colonizing the subject: The politics of gender in women's autobiography* (pp. 91–114). Minneapolis: University of Minnestoa Press.

Bion, W. R. (1961/1989). *Experiences in groups and other papers*. New York: Brunner-Routledge.

Blechner, M. (2014). Dissociation among psychoanalysts about sexual boundary violations. *Contemporary Psychoanalysis*, *50*(1): 1–11.

Boulanger, G. (2012). Psychoanalytic witnessing: Professional obligation or moral imperative? *Psychoanalytic Psychology*, *29*(3): 318–324.

Bromberg, P. (1998). *Standing in the spaces: Essays on clinical process, trauma and dissociation*. New York: Routledge.

Butler, J. (1997). *The psychic life of power: Theories in subjection*. Stanford, CA: Stanford University Press.

Celenza, A. (2007). *Sexual boundary violations: Therapeutic, supervisory, and academic contexts*. Lanham, MD: Aronson.

Cornell, D. (2010). The ethical affirmation of human rights: Gayatri Spivak's intervention. In R. C. Morris (Ed.), *Reflections on the history of an idea: Can the subaltern speak?* (pp. 100–114). New York, NY: Columbia University Press.

Daly, K. (2006). Restorative justice and sexual assault. *British Journal of Criminology*, *46*: 334–356.

Davies, J. M. & Frawley, M. G. (1992). Dissociative processes and transference countertransference paradigms in the psychoanalytically oriented treatment of adult survivors of childhood sexual abuse. *Psychoanalytic Dialogues*, *2*: 5–36.

Dekeseredy, W. & Kelly, K. (1993). The incidence and prevalence of woman abuse in Canadian university and college dating relationships. *Canadian Journal of Sociology*, *18*: 137–159.

Dimen, M. (2011). Lapsus linguae, or a slip of the tongue?: A sexual violation in an analytic treatment and its personal and theoretical aftermath. *Contemporary Psychoanalysis*, *47*: 35–79.

Douglas, M. (1966). *Purity and danger*. New York: Routledge.

Doyle, J. (2015). *Campus sex Campus security.* Semiotext(e) intervention series 19. Boston, MA: MIT Press.

Elise, D. (2015). Unraveling: Betrayal and the loss of goodness in the analytic relationship. *Psychoanalytic Dialogues, 25*(5): 557–571.

Faimberg, H. (2005). *Telescoping of generations: Listening to the narcissistic links between generations.* London: Routledge.

Feldmen, S. & Laub, D. (1992). *Testimony: Crises of witnessing in literature, psychoanalysis, and history.* NY: Routledge.

Foehl, J. C. (2005). "How could this happen to me?": Sexual misconduct and us. *Journal of the American Psychoanalytic Association, 53*(3): 957–970.

Gentile, K. (2013a). Biopolitics, trauma and the public fetus: An analysis of preconception care. *Subjectivity, 6*(2): 153–172.

———. (2013b). Bearing the cultural in order to engage in a process of witnessing. *Psychoanalytic Psychology, 30*(3): 456–470.

———. (2015). Generating subjectivity through the creation of time. *Psychoanalytic Psychology, 33*(2): 264–283.

———. (2017a). Chasing justice: Bystander intervention and restorative justice in the contexts of college campuses and psychoanalytic institutes. In K. Davisson & E. Toronto (Eds.), *A womb of her own.* Section III of Division 39. London: Karnac Books.

———. (2017b). Collectively creating conditions for emergence. In S. Grand & J. Salzberg (Eds.), *Wounds of history: Transgenerational trauma.* New York: Routledge.

———. (2018). Assembling justice: Reviving nonhuman subjectivities to address institutional betrayal around sexual misconduct. *Journal of the American Psychoanalytic Association, 66* (4): 647–678.

Gentile, K., Raghavan, C., Rajah, V., & Gates, K. (2007). It doesn't happen here?: Eating disorders in an ethnically diverse sample of low-income, female and male, urban college students. *Eating Disorders: The Journal of Treatment and Prevention, 15*(5): 405–425.

Gerson, S. (2009). When the third is dead: Memory, mourning, and witnessing in the aftermath of the Holocaust. *International Journal of Psychoanalysis, 90*: 1341–1357.

Grand, S. (2002). Between the reader and the read: Commentary on paper by Elizabeth F. Howell. *Psychoanalytic Dialogues, 12*(6): 959–970.

Grand, S. (2003). Unsexed and ungendered bodies: The violated self. *Studies in Gender and Sexuality, 4*(4): 313–341.

Herman, C. M. (2012). Sex with patient caused no harm, doctor says. *CommonWealth: Policitcs, Ideas, & Civic Life in Massachusetts.* January 26, 2012. Downloaded September, 2013.

Honig, R. G. & Barron, J. W. (2013). Restoring institutional integrity in the wake of sexual boundary violations: A case study. *Journal of the American Psychoanalytic Association, 61*(5): 897–924.

Kasper, B. (2004). Campus-based women's centers: Administration, structure and resources. *NASPA Journal, 41*(3): 487–489.

Koss, M. P., Wilgus, J. K., & Williamsen, K. M. (2014). Campus sexual misconduct: Restorative justice approaches to enhance compliance with Title IX guidance. *Trauma, Violence, & Abuse, 15*(3): 42–257.

Layton, L. (2010). Irrational exuberance: Neoliberal subjectivity and the perversion of the truth. *Subjectivity, 3*: 303–322.

Levin, C. (2014). Trauma as a way of life in a psychoanalytic institute. In R. A. Deutsch (Ed.), *Traumatic ruptures: Abandonment and betrayal in the analytic relationship* (pp. 176–196). New York and London: Routledge.

Levine, H. B. (2010a). Sexual boundary violations: A psychoanalytic perspective. *British Journal of Psychotherapy, 26*(1): 50–63.

———. (2010b). The sins of the fathers: Freud, narcissistic boundary violations and their effects on the politics of psychoanalysis. *International Forum of Psychoanalysis, 19*: 43–50.

Mackler, D. (2006). An analysis of the shadow side of Frieda Fromm-Reichmann. *International Society for Psychological & Social Approaches to Psychosis Newsletter, 7*(1), 10–12.

Margalit, A. (2002). *The ethics of memory.* Cambridge, MA: Harvard University Press.

Mitchell, S. A. (2000). *Relationality: From attachment to intersubjectivity.* New York: Routledge.

Mohanty, C. T. (2004). *Feminism without borders: Decolonizing theory, practicing solidarity.* Durham, NC: Duke University Press.

Morrison, S., Hardison, J., Mathew, A., & O'Neil, J. (2004). *An evidence-based review of sexual assault preventive intervention programs.* Washington: National Institute of Justice.

Oliver, K. (2001). *Witnessing: Beyond recognition.* Minneapolis, MN: University of Minnesota Press.

Oliver, K. (2004). *The colonization of psychic space: A psychoanalytic social theory of oppression.* Minneapolis, MN: University of Minnesota Press.

Poland, W. S. (2000). The analyst's witnessing and otherness. *Journal of the American Psychoanalytic Association, 48*: 17–34.

Ruskin, R. (2011). Sexual boundary violations in a senior training analyst: Impact on the individual and psychoanalytic society. *Canadian Journal of Psychoanalysis, 19*(1): 87–106.

Saketopoulou, A. (2010). Consent, sexuality, and self-respect: Commentary on Skerrett's "beyond consent". *Studies in Gender and Sexuality, 12*: 245–250.

Skerrett, K. R. (2010). Beyond "consent": David Mamet's *Oleanna* and a hostile environment for souls. *Studies in Gender and Sexuality, 12*: 235–244.

Smith, C. P. & Freyd, J. J. (2014). Institutional betrayal. *American Psychologist, 69*(6): 575–587.

Spivak, G. C. (1988). Can the subaltern speak? In C. Nelson & L. Gorssberg (Eds.), *Marxism and the interpretation of culture* (pp. 271–313). Basingstoke, UK: Macmillan Education.

Sue, D. W., Capodilupo, C. M., Torino, G. C., Bucceri, J. M., Holder, A. M. B., Nadal, K. L., & Esquilin, M. (2007). Microaggressions in everyday life: Implications for clinical practices. *American Psychologist, 62*(4): 271–286.

Tronto, J. C. (1994). *Moral boundaries: A political argument for an ethic of care.* New York: Routledge.

Ullman, C. (2006). Bearing witness: Across the barriers in society and in the clinic. *Psychoanalytic Dialogues, 16*: 181–198.

Wallace, E. M. (2007). Losing a training analyst for ethical violations: A candidate's perspective. *International Journal of Psychoanalysis, 88*: 1275–1288.

White, J. W. & Koss, M. P. (1991). Courtship violence: Incidence in a national sample of higher education students. *Violence and Victims, 6*: 247–256.

Chapter 6

Does the sexual have anything to do with sexual boundary violations?

Avgi Saketopoulou

In this paper I describe two sexual boundary violations that were alleged to have occurred in my analytic institute while I was still a candidate. While there is no way of ascertaining with certainty the veracity of those allegations,[1] the rumors around them produced tremendous distress and confusion in my community. As is common in these situations, the feelings evoked were amplified by the fact that neither the rumored breaches nor the institutional responses to them were openly discussed or processed. Drawing on my observations of the affects they engendered in my colleagues and in myself, I offer three sets of propositions regarding our collective relationship to sexual boundary violations. I start with an introductory summary to the ideas I will be exploring and proceed to a detailed description of what I understood to have transpired in my institute. I then take a step back to pursue a set of theoretical ideas regarding the neglected role of sexuality in the matter of sexual infractions. At the end of the essay, I return to the alleged incidents and to an enactment that also occurred at my institute at that same time to offer some propositions that may further our understanding of sexual breaches in the consulting room.

Erotic countertransference as erotic risk: three implications

Erotic and sexual feelings are always a possibility when two people spend considerable amounts of time together. Possibility becomes likelihood when this proximity occurs under conditions architected to promote intimacy, as is the case in psychoanalytic treatments. Further augmenting the probability that the analyst may experience feelings of erotic love towards an analysand is the fact that the psychoanalyst's office, in both its privacy and its epiphenomenal excitements, lends itself to the illusion that, if only in 45-minute instalments, our patients belong to us. Psychoanalysis should have much to say about how ordinary and even how expectable it may be for erotic affect to germinate in the analyst. But it does not. While we have a very developed discourse around the prevalence of the patient developing romantic or sexual feelings towards her treating analyst, speaking to the analyst's sexual and in-love feelings has proven to be incredibly challenging. For the most part, we tend to overlook how pervasive, expectable and incredibly difficult such countertransferences may be for the analyst *on the personal level.*

There exists, of course, a vast analytic literature on erotic countertransference. But this literature, I propose, is insufficient because it speaks of the analyst's erotic attractions as an *iatrogenic phenomenon* and, further, because it does so in flat and aseptic language. Lacking frankness and honesty, it neglects the embodied dimension of some erotic countertransferences and most often does not convey the arresting force with which it can take hold of the analyst (for rare exceptions see Ceccoli, 2015; Elise, 2015). In large part, we refrain from speaking about the force of erotic countertransference because of how frightening it is to acknowledge that we are all exquisitely vulnerable to boundary violations (Celenza, 2007) *and that this vulnerability is endemic to the practice of our craft.* Such an acknowledgement would have us face the fact that embodied and sexual risks are *structural* to the treatment situation, that we are always and from the start in a precarious position vis-à-vis our analysands.

On the collective level we try to manage our discomfort around the sexual and erotic risks that inhere in all treatments by talking about erotic countertransference in largely de-sexualised ways. As a result, our conversations regarding the analyst's erotic feelings tend to be flat, not reflecting the agitated intensity that can accompany the stirring of sexual desire. In a rather banal sense, erotic countertransference is, in fact, treated no differently than psychoanalysis has been treating the metapsychology of all sexuality (Dimen, 1999; Green, 1995). Relocated from post-oedipal embodied relation into pre-oedipal de-sexualized attachment, the sexual is nowadays mostly mined for object relational meanings (Fonagy, 2008). But exclusive attribution of the analyst's erotic feelings to the set of interpersonal object relational dynamics activated in the dyad[2] over-looks how, as clinicians, we also have to contend with our own sexual embodiment, with erotic passion and with the temptations of erotic surrender. This de-sexualization of erotic countertransference aug-ments our risk for boundary violations in three different ways:

1. Sterilized portrayals of erotic countertransference erase the vigor and phenomenological intensity of the experience, leaving ana-lysts who are caught in the powerful undertow of eros vulner-able to the defensive rationalization that their experience is somehow unique or fundamentally different from that of their colleagues. Comparing one's powerfully embodied response to a patient to blunted descriptions of erotic countertransference in the analytic literature can lead an analyst to conclude that their experience is exceptional. Drawing a distinction between *real* versus *countertransference love* is not only conceptually mistaken (transference and countertransference phenomena are not any less "real" than extra-analytic experiences); it is dangerous. It is dangerous because when swayed by such rationalizations, an analyst may be tempted to conclude that since their feelings are "real" it is legitimate to act on them, thereby capsizing an ana-lysis into a sexual violation.[3]

2. While on a conscious level we staunchly and definitively con-demn sexual relations with patients, on the level of the uncon-scious we are more conflicted and ambivalent than we want to believe. In fantasy, our patients are always potential sexual objects and possible erotic or romantic partners. Ensuring that these fantasies do not become acted out requires a certain amount of psychic work.[4] This work involves the labor of relin-quishing our unconscious sexual claims on our patients and cannot be accomplished on a cognitive level. It requires more than dutiful submission to the ethical proscriptions of our pro-fession. Part of that labor no doubt belongs to our individual treatments. But another part of it, and this will be the second point in my essay, can *only* be accomplished on the level of the

group. It involves a shift in our engagement around erotic countertransference so that it no longer erases the fact that the work
of analysis produces the very conditions under which analysts
may develop erotic feelings towards their patients. And it
requires that the group be able to tolerate and not pathologize
the intensity with which these feelings can develop in the analyst. If we can't bear to know that our work opens up the possibility that one may develop enthralling erotic passions about her
patient, how will we carry out ourselves and help others carry
out the psychic labor involved in relinquishing these desires?

3.   Last, I will suggest that our profession's anxious inability to
acknowledge the erotic risk inherent in the treatment situation cultivates a dense nexus of unspeakable erotic affect, of disavowed
embodied longing, of split-off sexual arousal and of disowned
romantic fantasy. This affective cloud is a property of the
collective.[5] It is mired in excess (Stein, 2008) and traffics in unformulated states (Stern, 2003). This cloud creates certain kinds of
larger scale psychic pressures to which some analysts may be more
vulnerable than others. From this angle, the transgressing analyst
can be understood as the particular subject where the collective
pressures of unacknowledged, unmourned and unrelinquished
erotic tensions come to hatch. Hartman (2013) has used the term
risk object to describe how some subjects become lightning rods
for the expression of unbearable group affect and I use his work to
flesh out how these ideas might be useful in furthering our understanding of transgressors.

This focus, obviously, does not mean to imply that the transgressing
analyst be exonerated or that her undeniable personal responsibility
in the case of a sexual violation be negated. And, as Gabbard
(1994a, 1994b) and Gabbard and Lester (1995) have pointed out,
some analysts may be more vulnerable to acting out due to personal
and situational factors. I am only hoping to add a consideration of
larger scale group dynamics to this topic using Muriel Dimen's
(2016) brilliant insistence on sexual boundary violations as being
also "a problem of the group". From her new and original perspective, sexual abuses in the consulting room cannot be sufficiently
addressed by attending only to individual or dyadic factors:

interventions on the level of psychoanalysis as a field and as a discipline are necessary. Revamping our literature on erotic countertransference to reflect the embodied dimensions of the experience and having more open and honest conversations about the necessity *and* the difficulty of renouncing our patients as sexual objects are vital in the effort to dispel as much as possible the intricate and insidious force of our shared ambivalence. These interventions have to start early in analytic training and in my closing remarks I offer concrete suggestions as to what may be helpful to address. It is important to note, however, that frank and open discussions about erotic countertransference need to continue *throughout* the analyst's professional life. I hope that this paper helps explain why doing so can be an act of collective self-care (see also Harris, this volume) that may function as an exoskeleton to protect some analysts from sexual acting out.

Invitation to write

When Dr. Charles Levin approached me about contributing a chapter to a volume inspired by Dimen's classic *Lapsus Linguae* (2011), I felt a surge of enthusiasm, then agitation.

My enthusiasm drew on my sense that space had been pried open by Dimen's call to psychoanalysts to rethink how we engage the enduring problem of sexual abuses in clinical praxis. Dimen effectively re-wrote the discursive protocols for this very tortured topic and did so by speaking from both sides of the couch, as both analyst and analysand. Dimen not only told us but, more importantly, she *showed* us by means of her dexterously theorized personal narrative the importance of not turning a deaf ear to the thudding "sound of silence" (Dimen, 2011, p. 39) around sexual infractions. These silences, she insisted, occur under the auspices of massive denial and dissociation, processes that frequently underwrite sexual transgressions and that manifest in the analyst/analysand dyad as well as on the institutional level (Ruskin, 2011; Wallace, 2007).

At the same time, Dr. Levin's invitation to write about psychosexual boundary violations came at a time during which my analytic institute had been reeling from a series of events that were rumored to involve some version or another of a sexual breach. Therefore, the prospect of writing this chapter soaked me in anxiety. Allegations that I'll describe shortly were met with a striking and painful absence of communal discussion. Noting that the roster of analysts invited to contribute to this volume drew heavily from my institute's community (which was also Muriel Dimen's), I wondered – perhaps fantasized – whether this volume might become the symbolic space where the range of conversations we were unable to have in the institutional frame could finally be hosted.[6] In sharing these anonymized allegations as I understood them I am joining others before me who have felt that they are "revealing well-guarded family secrets" (Gabbard & Peltz, 2001, p. 660).

Two boundary violations and an enactment

Just as Dimen's freshly published paper *Lapsus Linguae* was beginning to break ground, an allegation of a sexual transgression came forth in my institute. A widely respected and admired senior faculty member was said to have become erotically involved with a patient. Some of my colleagues seemed to have "insider information," but for the majority of our membership, rumor and gossip fed the ensuing pandemonium of behind-the-scenes conversations. Feelings of alarm, disbelief and discomfort fueled the fast-spreading speculation and with each round of re-telling, misunderstanding and misremembering accrued. Fantasy and projection rushed in with further embellishments, generating more tumult and added turmoil.

There was much conjecture as to the length of the analysis the transgression had ruptured (for some analysts, a short consultation seemed to mitigate the harm to the patient); whether it pertained to an ephemeral sexual liaison or to an enduring romantic relationship that would lead to marriage (to some the latter legitimated the boundary violation[7]); and last, but certainly not least, questions about what would be the fate of the transgressing analyst's institutional affiliations, supervisory responsibilities and leadership positions.

The horde of questions with which we were becoming preoccupied called for answers. This seeking of information was also an attempt to bind affect, primarily anxiety; if we could "understand" what happened, something would feel more settled – or so the implicit promise went. Primitive defenses fueled the buzz of disbelief that ensued. Traumatic experience, Eigen writes, "counts on the time lapse ... between the horror that leads to disbelief, and the horror that awakens realization of one's condition" (2007, p. 77). Disbelief and horror abounded indeed. How could *this* particular analyst, well-trained and respected in our community, be identified as a potential transgressor (read denial: aren't good analysts exempt from such gross acting out)? Might the analyst in question have been caught in a psychotic transference (read splitting: good analyst/bad patient)? Was the patient perhaps overly seductive (read disavowal: perhaps sexual acting had occurred but was not, ultimately, the analyst's fault)? What were the implications for institute members who had been taught and/or supervised and/or treated by this person (read contagion (Dimen, 2001; this volume)): is this a "defect" that might have been passed onto his supervisees, analysands and students)? How could this have happened in *our* institute (read idealization: weren't *we* better trained/analyzed/aware of countertransference issues than colleagues in "those" institutes where transgressions were known to have occurred)?

With more candidates, graduates and faculty joining the conversation, the matter of how the institute would address this problem became increasingly urgent. My institute functions under university auspices and this raised several previously unanticipated difficulties. For instance, could an investigation issue from our Ethics committee or would it have to be handled by the university administration and be, thus, driven by a different set of legal considerations? Word of mouth and eventually more formal communications cautioned us that serious legal ramifications in the form of potential libel suits might await those who spoke with names or information that could be – or be seen as – identifying.[8] The stakes of a legal suit were not insignificant. But I was incredulous that legal advice so matter-of-factly clashed with our analytic valuation of open conversation. I also shared my colleagues' worry that these interdictions to speech would exacerbate the situation. And of course, while some of the silences that ensued were enforced by legal advice and its paranoid amplifications, dissociation also had its heyday.[9]

Who knew what and in how much detail depended on whether one had personal relations with those "in the know" and/or access to investigations/complaints, as opposed to whether one heard about these events through the formal and carefully worded communications from our institute's administration. Each degree of separation marked decreased access, which set up an information – and chatter – hierarchy with gradations of "insiders" and "outsiders" (Grossmark, 2017). Our community, it felt to me, began to fragment. Loyalties to the training analyst/beloved teacher in question also split us into groups with differing priorities; to protect the analyst's reputation; to pronounce the truthfulness/falsity of the allegation; to express concern for the patient's welfare; to voice worry for our institute's integrity and reputation. Each set of responses seemed to hold onto parts of a whole that could not be integrated (on this dynamic see also, Ruskin, 2011).

Gossip, the dialect of unmetabolized affect, escalated quickly, generating a field that vibrated in radioactive intensity.[10] Soon, another story started circulating. It went somewhat like this: one of the candidates in the next academic year's incoming class was married to her former analyst. It was unclear whether the relationship had started pre- or post-termination, and if so by how long. As the patient in that treatment, the prospective candidate of course bore no ethical responsibility for the breach. Nor were any explanations owed to anyone about the candidate's personal choices. From an institutional viewpoint, nevertheless, there was a remarkable, even if un-remarked upon, contradiction: on the one hand lay the ordinary analytic proscription against erotic relations with patients. On the other hand, one of our new colleagues' life conditions now spoke vociferously – and with the institutional legitimacy of marriage – from across the divide of sexual boundary violations. And this contradiction "happened" to become concretized in our midst at this particular moment when a potential transgression by a respected colleague was actively preoccupying us.

One could think of this odd decision to accept this candidate into training as an unrelated coincidence. But to me, this kind of administrative choice made at *this* particular moment seemed overdetermined. Materializing at a time and in a milieu already suffering from the sequelae of a possible sexual infraction, it felt to be more enactment than accident. As a private matter, the candidate's marriage ought to be respected and, thus, not be an object of gossip. As such, the institutional decision could not be openly discussed and no feelings could be aired. The situation became embedded with confusion to the point where the conflicting messages coming from the Institute to the membership could not be clearly identified. Some assumed that this institutional gesture and the silence around it, which compounded the traumatic silence around the alleged violation, must be saturated with unconscious meanings. Questions began to emerge around what belonged in the sphere of the private and what, as a matter that affected the whole membership, might be seen as pertaining to the public domain.

A mere six months later new rumors started spreading. They alleged a new sexual transgression. The grapevine spoke of a young colleague who had been previously regarded as extremely promising and very talented. A renewed surge of high-voltage speculation about the parameters of the violation, possible institutional responses, etc., quickly followed. This was feeling like a bad joke: "history repeats" wrote Marx, "first as tragedy, then as farce" (1852, p. 1). The second allegation and its investigation caused an even bigger institutional crisis that culminated in the resignation of our Ethics committee. The disbandment was followed by a series of well-intended, thoughtfully composed but nevertheless cryptic communications from institute administration. On the one hand candidates, graduates and faculty were strongly encouraged to discuss the matter openly with each other. On the other hand, we were also informed that for legal reasons such conversations could not be organized by or include the institute's administration; they could not involve the sharing of investigative information or provisional findings; they could not be held on the institute's physical premises; and they could not involve use of the institute resources (e.g. our online listserve). Our Ethics committee has since been reinstated: its newly defined mission is exclusively educational.

With other members of our analytic community, I was shaken by these two allegations of transgressions occurring in such rapid succession and I was confused as to how to understand the admission of a candidate married to their former analyst in the midst of these unfolding crises. In the remainder of this essay, I explore several formulations regarding clinical sexual abuses and their relevance to what I understand to have occurred in my institute.

Theory, practice, risk

Theoretical and clinical psychoanalysis part ways precisely on the issue of risk. In the *written word* psychoanalysis is a set of brilliant and revolutionary ideas which, when wielded with equal measures of intelligence and courage, reveal that seemingly mundane coincidences, errors, repetitions, slips and dreams are, in fact, saturated with meaning; that the manifestly irrational gets two votes when reason gets only one; that temporality works backwards and laterally as well and as often as it works in time-forward; that psychic life is a delicate and complex encounter between inner and outer, self and other, family and the State.

But in the *intersubjective flesh*, clinical psychoanalysis is the inter-embodied (Hartman, 2010) practice of sitting dyadically, albeit asymmetrically, with different kinds of risk, at times even inviting it: regressions risk breakdown; dependence risks primitive terror; transference risks idealization, hatred and envy; intimacy risks being missed or, more difficult yet, being known.

Assuming these kinds of risks is indispensible to our clinical method. Without them psychoanalysis depreciates from valuable tool to mere intellectual exercise. It is through their valiant engagement, which can only materialize against a backdrop of relative and always illusory safety (Levy & Inderbitzin, 1997), that the work of psychoanalysis acquires its therapeutic traction. As analysts we make it our business to keep these perils in mind even when – *if not especially because* – we can't always anticipate them. We make it our business to safeguard our ability to think despite their fracturing pressures and we do so in the interest of deepening, mourning, experiencing, and freeing. And indeed, in our clinical literature and in our theories of technique we speak about these risks well and often. But we rarely acknowledge the ubiquity of the erotic risks that inhere in the practice of our craft. In fact, while the topic of risk has been taken up in the literature on boundary violations (e.g. Margolis, 1997; Pinsky, 2011), to my knowledge analytic scholarship has not recognized that the *erotic* dimension of the risks endemic to the analytic situation for the analyst.

Consider, for example, Adam Phillips' description of psychoanalysis as "what two people can say to each other if they agree to not have sex" (quoted in Bersani & Phillips, 2008, p. 1). Even when made between parties operating under the well-intentioned promise that one person will, for the most part, bracket their own needs to attend to the other's, such interpersonal agreements sometimes *do* fail. One promises but one doesn't always deliver. And since promises and commitments are liens on the future, their dependability can only be assessed in reversed time.

For an analyst, then, to believe with unshakeable certainty in her promise to her patients that sexual boundaries will not be crossed, requires the help of some naïve optimism, if not downright self-deception (Gabbard, 2008; Gabbard & Hobday, 2012). This is not only because the unconscious can make fools of us all. It is also because the disciplinary commitment necessary to deliver on Phillips' pledge requires that we relinquish our patients as possible sexual object choices. How, however, can we do that if we cannot bear to acknowledge in the first place that the analyst might develop untameable sexual desires towards her patients? Renouncing them (by which I mean not eliminating but not acting on them), requires more of us than the obligatory, intellectualized repetitions of the proscription against sexual contact. It requires processing loss, so that loss may become grievable.

In the absence of such emotional processing, our overall relationship to sexual contact with patients remains enduringly ambivalent and conflicted. Perhaps emblematic of that ambivalence is the observation that suspicions – let alone the fact – of sexual boundary transgressions tend to command widespread states of excited agitation and of ecstatic horror. The alarm and tumult of sexual infractions becomes quickly compelling and the gossip accompanying rumors of such occurrences is oftentimes animated and sensationalized. Powerful identifications and defensive counter-identifications fuel the unending cascades of rumors that entwine voyeuristic pleasure and horror (Slochower, 2017). When transgression is encountered, we are not just appalled. We are pumped up, we are energized and fascinated. This should give us all pause.

The psychic work of renunciation

Psychoanalysis has traditionally conceptualized the work of renunciation through a developmental paradigm. For Klein (1946) that psychic process requires the immeasurably difficult transition from the omnipotence of the paranoid-schizoid position to the excruciating admission of one's own limits. Genuinely relinquishing control over the object is a precondition for true mourning and for the move into depressive functioning. For Klein, as well as for more contemporary

Kleinians (Steiner, 2011), this is a lifelong, one-person struggle. But from the more relational perspective of Loewald (1979) this is a two-person job: not only the child, but the caretaker too must give up a narcissistic fantasy of considerable appeal if an oedipal resolution is to be achieved. The parent's cooperation is critical in this path to psychic emancipation because the parent has to allow herself to be relocated from her child's center stage to the periphery, to accept, that is, to be dethroned – a process that Loewald likened to parenticide. Relational authors have picked up this theoretical baton, stretching these ideas beyond considerations of power and emancipation but also to the dynamics of eroticism (Cooper, 2003; Davies, 1994, 1998, 2001, 2003, 2004, 2013). Oedipus, Davies writes, is "really not the child's complex but, at least when it goes wrong ... [it is about] the parent's inability to let the child move [on] ..." (in Slavin, Oxenhandler, Seligman, Stein & Davies, 2004, p. 395).[11]

This dynamic resurfaces in the analytic situation during termination, the ultimate relinquishment of our patients if ever there was one (Davies, 2010). In the termination phase, enactments around the renunciation of the patient as *ours* play out in the most primitive ways and with extraordinary urgency (Salberg, 2010a, 2010b). It is no accident, thus, that the risk of the analyst's sexual acting out is especially heightened during that period (Gabbard, 1994b). Sexual breaches in treatment may be intimately connected with the analyst's difficulty in relinquishing the analysand as a potential object of *sexual or romantic relations.*

How the erotic countertransference omits the register of sexuality

There is a striking, though rather ordinary, omission in my narration of what seems to have transpired at my institute. My description engaged matters of ethics, truth, anxiety, rules, responsibility, horror, scapegoating, legalities, loyalty, privacy, information hierarchies and so on. Other than in the naming of the boundary transgression as sexual in nature, nowhere is sexuality's key role acknowledged. This omission, as I mentioned, is not at all unusual. It is actually quite common that discussions of and scholarship about putative sexual infractions focuses on intersubjective dynamics and on institutional impact and/or institutional response (Gabbard & Lester, 1995; Wallace, 2007). On the role of sexuality in such infractions, psychoanalysis is selectively mute. And here is the paradox to which I want to call our attention: sexual contact is the problem we are struggling with *yet the matter of the sexual is strikingly absent from our discourse on it*! Refusing to consider how the sexual bears on this issue does not make it go away, it just sends our awareness of it underground. And by doing so it defines differently the terms by which we engage the sexual in the consulting room: through disavowal, that perfect psychic precondition of acting out. We need to wonder then: *Does the sexual really have nothing to do with sexual infractions?*

Most psychoanalytic conversations about the role of sexuality in the analytic setting tend to focus on how and when to talk to patients about sex. This is no doubt an important and thorny technical issue. Because language is always already enactive, because it performatively "materializes what it aims to describe" (Goldner, 2003, p. 120), we have to be mindful that when speaking with analysands about sexuality words are not entirely on our side. This muddies the line between intimate speech and sexual engagement. How does one talk about *being* turned on without someone *getting* turned on? Further complicating matters is that speaking about sexuality is also layered with enigmatic communications (Laplanche, 1987), with unconscious meaning and unconscious fantasy that by definition elude the speaker's consciousness. As such, the shame, disgust, seduction, arousal, inhibition, excitement and fear that swirl through sexual talk (Stein, 2008) are easily downloaded from patient to analyst and vice versa. As these affects travel back and forth between analyst and analysand, their origin becomes difficult to locate and their precise effects hard to track. This is hopefully truer for the patient than it is for the analyst (Levine, 2010) but we understand that, to some degree, it is an eventuality for both members of the dyad.

Our disciplinary preoccupation, however, with *how* to speak with patients about sex seems to me to be also serving a defensive function. By focussing on questions of technique and of "how" to speak with patients about *their* sexual feelings, we consistently obscure that it is not only the patient's sexual subjectivity that is at stake but also that of the analyst. "The psycho-analyst" wrote Freud in his essay on transference love, "knows that he is working with highly explosive forces" (1915, p. 170). It appears to me, though, that we actually do not know that at all when it comes to the analyst. Our resistances to this kind of knowing are pervasive and insidious. There are vast differences between the intellectual sort of knowing that comes from absorbing facts and information on the cognitive level and the kind of knowing that happens on the level of *learning from experience*, what Bion called K (1984). This deeper knowing accrues as a result of painful psychic work; it involves feeling and being able to bear the sheer weight and the emotional impact of what it is we know.

Since it is part of our occupation to be "in the role of transference magnet on a stage *purposely tilted to court the patient's passion*" (Pinsky, 2011, p. 363), we should expect that many of us may, at some point, treat an analysand with whom we might have been lovers under different circumstances. We have yet to develop a professional culture facilitating this kind of conversation. Forensic discourse about sexual countertransference and sexual transgression has become part of our scientific tradition in recent decades (Cooper, 2016a, 2016b) but clinical discussions of sexual affects and feelings is not – at least not yet – in our canon. If we cannot speak to each other about how unremarkable it can be for an analyst to develop sexual or romantic feelings towards a patient, those who seek help by admitting to in-love and erotic feelings are discredited. And the rest of us get to imagine that the problem does not pertain to us (on the dynamic of the discreditable see also Dimen, 2016). Of course, public speech and writing about sex are difficult anyway, and speaking of sexual affects openly poses several problems. How, for instance, does one strike the right tone? How can we be frank but not salacious, descriptive and attentive to embodiment but not pornographic? These complicated issues need explicit and articulate attention and point to a discourse we very much need to develop.

The analyst's erotic and romantic feelings

We have no shortage of theories to account for the individual dynamics of the analytic transgressor. The analytic literature on sexual acting out is animated by theories around Oedipal rebellion, narcissism, rescue fantasies, borderline patients, power dynamics and differentials. But speaking of analysts' erotic desire per se continues to be especially vexed. This is especially true when it comes to the sexual body of the analyst or the analysand. Of sexual heat per se, of bodies and of feelings of being in love we routinely say very little. This is how disavowal becomes threaded into the discursive and professional reality of our field, birthing future analysts similarly unprepared for these conversations (Levin, 2014).

In order to consider the analyst's sexual body we have to take on the problem of its treacherous relationship to conscious life and its flagrant inattention to ethical principles. Against avowed plans and without our consent, our bodies may respond to those of our patients. These responses are not simply the aggregates of complex psychic states; they are embodied, lived experiences. Our physiological responses can be treacherous and disloyal: one does not control how one's heart rate quickens, how one's mouth dries out, how one's fingertips suddenly become more sensitive to sensation. At times, the analyst has to work from within such states of arousal, which is why it's so important that we be able to acknowledge the role of the sexual body as originator, as unwelcome instigator of experience, sometimes even as provocateur. Erotic affect, of course, is not only risk. It is, as we well know, analytic opportunity. It is only, however, if such experiences are carefully attended to, spoken about openly and perhaps even enjoyed, that the dynamically meaningful, somatically encoded information of erotic countertransferences may find their way into the analytic work. What would our discussions with each other look like if we spoke about erotic countertransference without unfastening it from the electrifying and destabilizing properties of sexuality?

In our literature, erotic countertransference becomes promptly unsexy, appearing only in the most dignified form – surely a defensive reaction formation to protect against the vigor and vitality of the experience. Even as pioneering analysts take up this issue, language is measured, even blunted. This makes erotic countertransference appear more clinically manageable and personally more controllable than it may, in fact, be. In this deceptively lighter, airier version erotic feelings get exclusively rerouted to the examination of psychodynamics, effectively divorced from passion and from the analyst's body.

Consider, for instance, Celenza's clinical report, where a patient whom she finds appealing confesses his attraction to her. In response, Celenza reports that she "smiled and felt a mutual resonant feeling" (2010, p. 180). Later on, with the help of the patient's confrontation, the analyst realizes that she has been distancing herself from him and through some self-analysis comes to realize that she has mobilized this distancing as a defense against the guilt of taking, perhaps, too much pleasure in her erotic countertransference. "[W]as I enjoying him too much?" she wonders courageously. And yet as readers, we have heard very little about what might have led the analyst to feel guilty, about the embodiment of her enjoyment or her possible sexual reverie: what we are told is that she experienced a "mutual resonant feeling" – a rather vague phrase. I am not suggesting that speaking differently would have been easy nor does Celenza more than any other analyst owe us an accounting that would involve exquisite vulnerability, not to mention unusual exposure. What I am pointing to, which Celenza also insists on reminding us, is that while *think* we want to talk about erotic feelings, doing so is astonishingly difficult (2010). The real impediments to speech, she argues, are unconscious. We are afraid. We are afraid of the psychoanalytic police, yes. But mostly we are afraid of ourselves. If an analyst who has worked extensively with boundary violators, and who has considered deeply matters of sexuality in the therapeutic situation (Celenza, 2014) – if *she* is wary of describing her erotic feelings even as she is forging new ground on that very topic, what chance do the rest of us have?

The chasm that exists between the phenomenology of such countertransferences, and the stilted language in which we speak of them, means that analysts who struggle with destabilizing erotic undercurrents in an analysis may not recognize themselves in the measured language of our analytic literature. In this context, analysts in the thrall of erotic longing may end up concluding that the intensity of their yearning is exceptional, that theirs is somehow "the real thing". Coming to believe that a reliable distinction can be drawn between countertransference love and "real love" can be an early warning sign of trouble (on this see also Celenza, 2015; 2021).

The notion that one's feelings are "real" can be the pivotal rationalization that tips the scales in the direction of a sexual transgression (Gabbard, 2008).

Psychoanalytic training

It has become commonplace to note that, as a discipline, we don't like to talk openly about the fact that sexual infractions occur in most institutes (Wallace, 2007), that they occur more often than we know or want to admit (Dimen, 2011), and that they will most likely continue to occur despite training and psycho-education (Celenza & Gabbard, 2003; Gabbard, 2016). While some of the psychic work necessary to minimize these possibilities belongs to our personal analyses, in this section I want to make some suggestions as to what analytic training can contribute to this process.

As I have been arguing, the de-sexualization of erotic countertransference can paradoxically end up subsidizing clinical sexual transgression. It's not that we don't know that erotic countertransferences can get out of hand. We even know that this is a problem to which we are all vulnerable (Celenza, 2007). What we do not know (in the Bionian, K sense of the term) is that the experiential dimension of these romantic and sexual states comes with the force of what Elise has described as a "riptide, catching one completely by surprise, overwhelming all efforts to swim toward shore. One minute you are fine, the next you're in the grip of a force so strong it cannot be combated with will" (2015, p. 288). This is a critical insight that analytic training should emphasize in order to prepare for the fact that overpowering erotic feelings may inhere in any psychoanalytic treatment. As importantly, training should alert us to the range of resistances we may encounter when it comes to relinquishing patients as potential sexual or romantic partners, forewarning us as to the range of defenses that can get unconsciously mobilized to prevent feelings of loss and from having to abdicate our sense of omnipotence over our patients – and ourselves.

Analysts should be trained to expect that under the pressure of erotic feelings, our understanding about the "as-if" nature of the transference may dissolve, setting the stage for the most vigorous rationalizations. Some analysts, for instance, may reason that these intense feelings are to be distinguished from clinical phenomena arising in the consulting room. Or, genuinely question whether a universal prohibition of sexual coupling with patients may be rigid or dated. From within such countertransferences' erotic tension, some may be tempted to argue that a patient's agency is to be respected[12] and that it may be infantilizing to question the patient's autonomous choices. Grandiose defenses may lead the analyst to consider her circumstances incomparable to everyone else's. She may then be inclined to isolate herself from her professional community convinced that her colleagues won't "understand", furthering the risk for a sexual violation.

It is important to note that since the analytic role requires us to remain permeable to our patients' psychic impact, we will not have at our disposal strategies of disengagement to which one ordinarily resorts in everyday interactions to ward off feelings that shouldn't be acted upon. The conscious strategies we all routinely employ to refrain from engaging in inappropriate sexual relationships can, therefore, not be mobilized in the clinical setting. As a result, the analyst may paradoxically find herself less equipped in the consulting room than she would be in everyday life to prevent acting out. Under these circumstances, staying true to her analytic role may be experienced as painful and be accompanied by feelings of loss. For some, this may incite anger or even hatred towards our profession (von Baeyer, 2013). All these factors should be conveyed to candidates as matters of course, integral to the meaning of dealing with erotic countertransferences, as expectable and unremarkable components of the experience.

Talking openly about the risks of erotic countertransference undoubtedly confronts us with extraordinary anxieties. That is made even more challenging by the fact that such acknowledgements render us exquisitely vulnerable to the outside world at a moment in time when attacks on psychoanalysis are at their most strident. One could easily imagine the discrediting uses to which such ideas might be put, how they could be levied against our clinical method. As if psychoanalysis did not have enough to tackle already regarding its public! Assuaging fears about erotic risk on the job is impossible because we cannot in full confidence point to a hard distinction between real love and transference or countertransference love. In actuality, Freud has instructed us (1915), all love is transferentially infused or, as Davies puts it, "there is indeed something between patient and analyst that is closer to other love relationships than we would like to believe" (in Slavin, Oxenahandler, Seligman, Stein & Davies, 2004, p. 397; see also Celenza, 2021; Schafer, 1993).

The analyst as risk object

I insist on highlighting that our personal analyses, our consultations with each other, our publications, our conferences and our professional conversations need to address embodied desire and erotic risk because I believe that erotics in the consulting room are not the exclusive purview of the dyad. Whereas it is true that any psychoanalytic treatment materializes between a single analyst and a single analysand, it is not, psychically speaking, a dyadic process. In addition to the internal object worlds of both, the analyst's mind also harbors an entire populace particular to her clinical work: her own analyst, her supervisors, her colleagues, her peers as well as an entire community of thinkers, theorists and clinicians, whose ideas, advice, cautionary notes and formulations are always active in the analyst's conscious and unconscious mind (Levine, 2010). And since it is in the nature of the psychoanalytic process to set up the conditions that may produce powerful erotic countertransferences and to then expect that the analyst forgo their acting out (Dimen, 2016, 2017), eroticism and its management is always already a property of the group.

As I have been discussing, our shared erasure of the analyst's erotic attractions to patients, and our lack of theorizing the process by which any possible sexual claims on our patients should be renounced heightens the risk for sexual breaches. To single out, then, the transgressing analyst as *the* site of sexual infraction is misguided. It may be helpful to think of the violating analyst as a *risk object* (Hartman, 2013), the host analyst into whom collective risk precipitates. The most vulnerable among us are, in some respects, the ventriloquists of our collective unspoken and unrelinquished eros. Desire, Hartman emphasizes, is not my excess – or yours – "[w]e are all in this together" (2013, p. 47). Surely we use the fallen to shore ourselves up, to assure ourselves that it is them and not us that are impure, contaminated, corrupt (Bataille, 1957; Douglas, 1966; Kristeva, 1982). But what I am suggesting here goes beyond thinking about scapegoating as an act of othering that works to rid itself of not-me aspects of self by righteously locating badness in the other. It is not just that the most vulnerable or the lovesick (Celenza, 2006; Twemlow & Gabbard, 1989) fall, but also that, on the level of the group, transgressors become the host objects where the disavowed force of our collective desire and our unmourned losses regarding sexual relations with patients may take up residence. Transgressors may be productively thought of as carriers of our communal ambivalence and of our unacknowledged erotic drive.

Two alleged sexual boundary violations and an enactment revisited

The reader may recall that the first allegation had been especially shocking because it named a senior and beloved faculty member. And yet, we might wonder about the assumptions inherent in that very concern: in other words, why would this analyst's level of experience and social regard in our community have the power to surprise us in the first place? I see that surprise as a symptom, indexing perhaps an underlying shared fantasy: We resort to considerations of the analyst's training, to the depth of his or her clinical experience and to how he or she is regarded in our professional communities as an indication of their clinical skill and ethical standing. Of course, none of these measures are good predictors of ethical conduct. But we rely on them because they offer the illusion of solidity against the overwhelming power that eroticism can wield in the consulting room. We levy them against eroticism's undertow in the hope that there are measurable qualities that can dependably dispel the power of sexual and in-love feelings.

Secondly, I see the timing of the admission of the candidate married to their former analyst as a dynamically significant enactment. On the level of unconscious group dynamics, this candidate served an important function: having been deputized to be the emblem of unacknowledged conflicts, of our active ambivalence about sexual relations with patients. Not exactly a full member, yet still part of the group, not precisely a scapegoat since the candidate is not expelled but "incorporated," the candidate became a means of binding the group's diffuse anxiety (activated by the first transgression), of absorbing as well as expressing our collective conflictual feelings, and of neutralizing its impact within the group. Candidates, because of their liminal status, as Levin (2014) has argued, are ideal material for being put to these kinds of object analytic institutes.

Third, I suggest that the knotted psychic space that formed in the mating of transgression, silence, and our disavowed ambivalence about sexual relations with patients, created the ideal conditions for our junior colleague to become a risk object. This colleague was a vulnerable conduit in whom the risk that our group could not hold or alphabetize (Ferro, 2002) manifested. Of course, I do not mean to mimimize this analyst's personal accountability; I am only trying to highlight that our collective ambivalence regarding sexual and romantic relations with patients manifests in individual analysts.

Closing remarks

To think of erotic countertransference as an ordinary risk that lives in all treatments disrupts our prized illusions of safety in the consulting room. In fact, the analyst's consulting room is one of the most dangerous places one can find oneself in. Revamping our regard for erotic countertransferences as not merely clinical phenomena but as expectable risks is necessary. Such a reconceptualization can help soften our grip on our idealized, false sense of safety and may permit us to absorb, and be better prepared psychically, for the fact that serious perils arise during a process that unfolds between two people in intimate contact whose psyches and whose embodiments can have reciprocally powerful impacts on each other. In that sense I agree with Dianne Elise (2015) that the nowadays-commonplace "slippery slope" metaphor that posits sexual transgressions as precipitated by a series of smaller non-sexual transgressions is a misnomer because it implies that with sufficient care and attention sexual infractions can be prevented. We would benefit from thinking about the analyst's sexual acting less as a series of graduated risks and more as a riptide that pulls us in with incredible force (Elise, 2015); a force the irresistibility of which is not easy to appreciate until one is caught in it; one which requires more than good training and solid ethics to sidestep; one which can be helped by a better functioning analytic group.

Notes

1 In the absence of an outright admission by the transgressing analyst, a conclusive investigation or a legal finding any rumor, claim, or allegation of a sexual boundary breach (whether true or false) has to be qualified as being an allegation rather than an event. See Gabbard (1999, 2008) and Gabbard and Peltz (2001) for a discussion of how this bears on how and how openly we can discuss such matters in our analytic institutes.
2 I am not, of course, proposing that such experiences are not highly significant or that they do not warrant serious clinical attention and care. The reader may consult works by Celenza (1998; 2010, 2011; this volume), Davies (2003, 2004) and Gabbard (1994a, 1994b, 2016) for highly nuanced discussions of these issues.
3 I am aware that a host of psychodynamics outside eroticism (disavowed rage, aggression, loss, envy, rescue fantasies etc.) have been identified as animating sexual infractions (see Celenza, 2007; Twemlow & Gabbard, 1989), but in this essay I want to focus on the neglected role of the erotic and in-love dimensions of such failed treatments.
4 Fantasies of sexual or romantic relations will always resurface and will do so, no doubt, at dynamically significant moments; the meanings of which need to be understood by the analyst.
5 I am using the term collective here to refer to an organized group that shares a sense of common goal, a group organized around a shared fantasy (Bion, 1961). One such shared fantasy in our profession is that as analysts we are always acting ethically and with our patients' best interests in mind.
6 A cadre of several analysts from my institute and from other NY-based institutes attempted to take on some of the problematics of silence following Dimen's (2011) paper by creating a conference to discuss these matters. These analysts included: Charles Amrhein, Mark Blechner, Velleda Ceccoli, Muriel Dimen, Katie Gentile, Adrienne Harris, Janine de Peyer, Sandy Silverman, Isaac Tylim, Jamieson Webster, and Cleonie White, as well as myself. Many dynamic – and some legal – issues that would require a paper unto itself to explicate and theorize, made it impossible to bring this project to fruition.
7 The fact that some such affairs survive the test of time has been used to argue in favor of the distinction between "transference love" and "real" love (on this see also Celenza, 2015; Schafer, 1977). To me this is problematic because it substitutes the question of the analyst's ethical responsibility with

an appeal to the institutional legitimacy and length of the subsequent relationship. Whether the consulting room can function as a good matchmak-
ing service is entirely beside the point. Further, the appeal to the possibility
of a "good marriage" overlooks that the psychoanalytic contract, as Guralnik (2021) aptly notes, is not only between analyst and patient, but also
between psychoanalysis and the public.

  8 Threats of litigation notoriously subtend the prohibition against talking
      about and taking action around issues of sexual acting out (Gabbard &
      Peltz, 2001; Ruskin, 2011). The legal defense against charges of libel is
      obviously the truth. However, the requirements for confidentiality and
      privacy particular to our profession make the "truth" nearly impossible
      to prove. This is especially so when the patient is not the complainant.
      Even in instances where one can successfully rebut libel suits, however,
      the fear of costly litigation effectively silences inquiry and speech.
  9 See Dimen (2016) for a discussion of dissociation's recalcitrant persist-
      ence when it comes to boundary violations.
 10 For further discussion of the traumatic impact of a sexual boundary
      violation on entire psychoanalytic communities, see Gabbard & Peltz,
      2001; Pinsky, 2011; Sandler & Godley, 2004; Wallace, 2007.
 11 It is important to be aware here that, while helpful, the often-drawn
      analogy between analyst/analysand and parent/child pairs also comes
      with significant limitations (see Davies, 2003).
 12 Though it is, of course, true that patients enter asymmetrical power
      relations all the time, the process of painstakingly architecting
      a relationship where regression and dependence unfurl is structural
      only to psychoanalysis.

References

Bataille, G. (1957). *Eroticism: Death and sensuality.* San Francisco: City
    Lights.
Bersani, L. & Phillips, A. (2008). *Intimacies.* Chicago: The University of Chi-
    cago Press.
Bion, W.R. (1961). *Experiences in groups and other papers.* London: Routledge.
Bion, W.R. (1984). *Learning from experience.* London: Karnac Books.
Ceccoli, V. (2015). *Paradise lost:* What is most dangerous about our method.
    Paper presented at the meeting of the International Association for Rela-
    tional Psychoanalysis, Toronto, June 24–28.
Celenza, A. (1998). Precursors to therapist sexual misconduct: Preliminary
    findings. *Psychoanalytic Psychology*, 15, 378–397.
Celenza, A. (2006). Sexual boundary violations in the office: When is
    a couch just a couch? *Psychoanalytic Dialogues*, 16(1), 113–128.

Celenza, A. (2007). *Sexual Boundary Transgressions: Therapeutic, Supervisory and Academic Contexts.* New York: Jason Aronson.

Celenza, A. (2010). The guilty pleasure of erotic countertransference: Searching for radial true. *Studies in Gender and Sexuality*, 11, 175–183.

Celenza, A. (2011). *Sexual boundary violations: Therapeutic, supervisory, and academic contexts.* New York: Jason Aronson.

Celenza, A. (2015). Lessons on or about the couch: What sexual boundary transgressions can teach us about everyday practice. Paper presented at the meeting of the International Association for Relational Psychoanalysis, Toronto, June 24–28.

Celenza, A. (2021). Shadows that corrupt: Present absences in the psychoanalytic process. In Levin, C. (Ed.) *Sexual Boundary Trouble in Psychoanalysis: Clinical Perspectives on Muriel Dimen's Concept of the "Primal Crime."* (pp. 77–93). New York and London.

Celenza, A. & Gabbard, G.O. (2003). Analysts who commit sexual boundary violations: A lost cause? *Journal of the American Psychoanalytic Association*, 51, 617–636.

Celenza, A. & Hilsenroth, M. (1997). Personality characteristics of mental health professionals who have engaged in sexualized dual relationships: A Rorschach investigation. *Bulletin of the Menninger Clinic*, 61, 90–107.

Cooper, S.H. (2003). You say oedipal, I say postoedipal. *Psychoanalytic Dialogues*, 13, 41–63.

Cooper, S.H. (2016a). Blurring boundaries or, why do we refer to sexual misconduct with patients as "boundary violation". *Psychoanalytic Dialogues*, 26(2), 206–214.

Cooper, S.H. (2016b). Reclaiming the boundary concept from forensic discourse: Response to commentaries. *Psychoanalytic Dialogues*, 26(2), 238–243.

Davies, J.M. (1994). Love in the afternoon: A relational reconsideration of desire and dread in the countertransference. *Psychoanalytic Dialogues*, 4(2), 153–170.

Davies, J.M. (1998). Between the disclosure and foreclosure of erotic transference-counter- transference: Can psychoanalysis find a place for adult sexuality? *Psychoanalytic Dialogues*, 8, 747–766.

Davies, J.M. (2001). Erotic overstimulation and the co-construction of sexual meaning in transference-countertransference experience. *Psychoanalytic Quarterly*, 70, 757–788.

Davies, J.M. (2003). Falling in love with love. *Psychoanalytic Dialogues*, 13, 1–27.

Davies, J.M. (2004). Whose bad objects are we anyway? Repetition and our elusive love affair with evil. *Psychoanalytic Dialogues*, 14, 711–732.

Davies, J.M. (2010). Transformations of desire and despair: Reflections on the termination process from a relational perspective. In Salberg, J. (Ed.), *Good enough endings: Breaks, interruptions, and terminations from contemporary relational perspectives* (pp. 109–130). New York, NY: Taylor & Francis.

Davies, J.M. (2013). My enfant terrible is twenty: A discussion of Slavin's and Gentile's retrospective reconsideration of "love in the afternoon". *Psychoanalytic Dialogues*, 23(2), 170–179.

Dimen, M. (1994). Money, love, and hate: Contradiction and paradox in psychoanalysis. *Psychoanalytic Dialogues*, 4(1), 69–100.

Dimen, M. (1999). Between *Lust* and Libido: Sex, Psychoanalysis, and the Moment Before. *Psychoanalytic Dialogues*, 9(4):415–440.

Dimen, M. (2001). Perversion is us? Eight notes. *Psychoanalytic Dialogues*, 11, 825–860.

Dimen, M. (2011). Lapsus linguae, or a slip of the tongue: A sexual violation in an analytic treatment and its personal and theoretical aftermath. *Contemporary Psychoanalysis*, 47(1), 35–79.

Dimen, M. (2016). Rotten apples and ambivalence: Sexual boundary violations through a psychocultural lens. *Journal of the American Psychoanalytic Association*, 64(2), 361–373.

Dimen, M. (2017). Eight topics: A conversation on sexual boundary violations between Charles Amrhein and Muriel Dimen. *Psychoanalytic Psychology*, 34(2), 169–174.

Douglas, M. (1966). *Purity and danger.* London: Routledge.

Eigen, M. (2007). *Feeling matters.* London: Karnac Books.

Elise, D. (2015). Psychic riptides: Swimming sideways: Reply to Dimen, Gabbard, and Harris. *Psychoanalytic Dialogues*, 25(5), 593–599.

Ferro, A. (2002). *Seeds of illness, seeds of recovery: The genesis of suffering and the role of psychoanalysis.* London: Routledge.

Fonagy, P. (2008). A genuinely developmental theory of sexual enjoyment and its implications for psychoanalytic technique. *Journal of the American Psychoanalytic Association*, 56, 11–36.

Freud, S. (1915). Observations on transference love. In Strachey, J. (Ed.), *The standard edition of the complete psychological works of Sigmund Freud* (vol. 12, pp. 157–171). London: Hogarth.

Gabbard, G.O. (1994a). On love and lust in erotic transference. *Journal of the American Psychoanalytic Asssociation*, 42, 385–403.

Gabbard, G.O. (1994b). Sexual excitement and countertransference love in the analyst. *Journal of the American Psychoanalytic Asssociation*, 42, 1083–1106.

Gabbard, G.O. (1999). Boundary violations and the psychoanalytic training system. *Journal of Applied Psychoanalytic Studies*, 1(3), 207–221.

Gabbard, G.O. (2008). Boundaries, technique and self-deception: A discussion of Arnold Goldberg's 'some limits of the boundary concept'. *Psychoanalytic Quarterly*, 77(3), 877–881.

Gabbard, G.O. (2016). Commentary on Steven Cooper's paper "blurring boundaries or, why do we refer to sexual misconduct with patients as 'boundary violations'". *Psychoanalytic Dialogues*, 26(2), 223–228.

Gabbard, G.O. & Lester, E.P. (1995). *Boundaries and boundary violations in psychoanalysis*. New York, NY: Basic Books.

Gabbard, G.O. & Peltz, M.L. (2001). Speaking the unspeakable: Institutional reactions to boundary violations by training analysts. *Journal of the American Psychoanalytic Association*, 49, 659–673.

Gabbard, G.S. & Hobday, G.O. (2012). A psychoanalytic perspective on ethics, self-deception and the corrupt physician. *British Journal of Psychotherapy*, 28(2), 235–248.

Goldner, V. (2003). Ironic gender/authentic sex. *Studies in Gender and Sexuality*, 4, 113–139.

Green, A. (1995) Has Sexuality Anything To Do With Psychoanalysis? (1995). *International Journal of Psycho-Analysis*, 76:871–883.

Grossmark, C. (2017). Candidates' responses to sexual boundary violations. *Psychoanalytic Dialogues*, 27(1), 79–88.

Guralnik, O. (2021). Sex and ethics. Protecting an enchanged space. In Levin, C. (Ed.), *Sexual Boundary Troiuble in Psychoanalysis: Clinical Perspectives on Muriel Dimen's Concept of the "Primal Crime."* (pp.94–104), New York and London: Routledge.

Hartman, S. (2010). Ruined by pleasure. *Studies in Gender and Sexuality*, 11, 141–145.

Hartman, S. (2013). Bondless love. *Studies in Gender and Sexuality*, 14, 35–50.

Klein, M. (1946). Notes on some schizoid mechanisms. *International Journal of Psychoanalysis*, 27, 99–110.

Kristeva, J. (1982). *Powers of horror*. New York: Columbia University Press.

Laplanche, J. (1987). *New foundations for psychoanalysis*. New York, NY: Blackwell.

Levin, C. (2014). Trauma as a way of life in a psychoanalytic institute. In Deutsch, R. (Ed.), *Traumatic ruptures: Abandonment and betrayal in the analytic relationship* (pp. 176–196). New York, NY: Routledge.

Levine, H.B. (2010). Sexual boundary violations: A psychoanalytic perspective. *British Journal of Psychotherapy*, 26(1), 50–63.

Levy, S.T. & Inderbitzin, L.B. (1997). Safety, danger and the analyst's authority. *Journal of the American Psychoanalytic Association*, 45, 377–394.

Loewald, H.W. (1979). The waning of the oedipus complex. *Journal of the American Psychoanalytic Association*, 27, 751–775.

Margolis, M. (1997). Analyst-patient sexual involvement: Clinical experiences and institutional responses. *Psychoanalytic Inquiry*, 17, 349–370.

Marx, K. (1852). *The eighteenth brumaire of Louis Bonaparte.* Berlin: Mondial.

Pinsky, E. (2011). The Olympian delusion. *Journal of the American Psychoanalytic Association*, 59, 351–375.

Ruskin, R. (2011). Sexual boundary violations in a senior training analyst: Impact on the individual and the psychoanalytic society. *Canadian Journal of Psychoanalysis*, 19(1), 87–106.

Salberg, J. (Ed.). (2010a). *Good enough endings: Breaks, interruptions, and termination from contemporary relational perspectives.* New York, NY: Routledge.

Salberg, J. (2010b). How we end: Taking leave. In Salberg, J. (Ed.), *Good enough endings: Breaks, interruptions, and terminations from contemporary relational perspectives* (pp. 109–130). New York, NY: Taylor & Francis.

Sandler, A. & Godley, W. (2004). Institutional responses to boundary violations: The case of Masud Khan. *International Journal of Psychoanalysis*, 85, 27–42.

Schafer, R. (1977). The interpretation of transference and the conditions of loving. *International Journal of Psychoanalysis*, 25, 335–362.

Schafer, R. (1993). Five readings of Freud's 'observations on transference-love'. In Person, E.S., Hagelin, A., & Fonagy, P. (Eds.), *On Freud's 'observations on transference-love'*, (pp. 75–95). New Haven: Yale University Press.

Slavin, J.H., Oxenhandler, N., Seligman, S., Stein, R., & Davies, J.M. (2004). Dialogues on sexuality in development and treatment. *Studies in Gender and Sexuality*, 5, 371–418.

Slochower, J. (2017, this volume). Don't tell anyone. *Psychoanalytic Psychology*, 34(2), 195–200.

Stein, R. (2008). The otherness of sexuality: Excess. *Journal of the American Psychoanalytic Association*, 56, 56–71.

Steiner, J. (2011). *Seeing and being seen: Emerging from a psychic retreat.* London: Routledge.

Stern, D.B. (2003). *Unformulated experience: From dissociation to imagination in psychoanalysis.* New York: Psychology Press.

Twemlow, S.W. & Gabbard, G. (1989). The lovesick therapist. In Gabbard, G. (Ed.), *Sexual exploitation in professional relationships* (pp. 71–87). New York, NY: American Psychiatric Publications.

von Baeyer, S. (2013). Sexual boundary violations: A hatred of psychoanalysis. Paper presented at the Wounds of History conference, New York, March 1–3.

Wallace, R. (2007). Losing a training analyst for ethical violations: A candidate's perspective. *International Journal of Psychoanalysis*, 88, 1275–1288.

Part III

Locating the psycho-sexual boundary

Chapter 7

Reflections on the aesthetics of the psychic boundary concept

Or, why refer to sexual misconduct with patients as boundary violation?[1]

Steven Cooper

For a number of years, I have been trying to figure out why the term *boundary violation* bothers me when used in reference to psychotherapists and psychoanalysts who engage in sexual relationships with their patients. With all due respect to my esteemed colleagues who are experts in the study of sexual misconduct (and I am not), I want to think through why referring to sexual misconduct and other ethical violations as *boundary* violations might be problematic. I will argue that our use of the term *boundary* for both psychic and behavioral realms has been obfuscating and detracts from the power of the boundary concept for understanding psychic phenomena.

In the art of psychoanalytic work, psychical boundaries are a process, not a thing. The process of analytic work involves trying to gain purchase on ways that patients and analysts play in the realm of psychic boundaries, including how these boundaries are understood and misunderstood. There is no such thing as a boundary but only various processes, intentions, and tendencies that generate the fiction or illusion or need for a boundary to be crossed or not crossed. I chaff against this "category confusion" because while there is no such *thing* as a psychic boundary, there is a line that cannot be crossed with reference to having sex with patients. I suggest that we make the term *boundary* into a kind of verb or participle in reference to talking about psychoanalytic work. Sexual activity is only a verb in reference to activity that is distinctly not psychoanalytic.

It is as if those who have developed the notion of ethical sexual misconduct are focusing in a more concrete way on the outposts of gross behavioral borders or boundaries but do not really address the density of boundary as an illusory, changing, developing phenomenon.

In relationship to psychic phenomena, boundaries are created rather than found. One of the many gifts of Winnicott's work (e.g. Winnicott, 1971) was to announce and continually elaborate for psychoanalysis how the act of finding and discovering are creative acts for patients and analysts. Lines between concrete and psychical, between reality and fantasy and even for love and hate are constantly interfused. In contrast to the imprecision of psychical boundaries, sexual misconduct is quite specific about lines that are distinct.

Sexual relationships with psychoanalytic patients are unethical. There are many reasons that analysts engage in sexual relationships with patients, and these have been well-explored by numerous authors (e.g., Celenza & Gabbard, 2003; Gabbard, 1994, 2008) and can be described in rich and specific ways depending on the psychological and emotional context in which this misconduct occurs.

We all think of boundaries in relation to the intrinsic complexity of psychic life—transference, fantasy, and the unconscious, as elaborated and lived out in the ritualized asymmetry of the psychoanalytic set-up. Part of the reason that I prefer to think about sexual misconduct in a language other than that of boundaries is related to aesthetics. For me, as a clinician, the aesthetics of the psychoanalytic arrangement, so utterly brilliant and complex, put more than enough on my plate about boundaries and borders. In referring to sexual activity with patients as a boundary issue, I believe we concretize and tame the concept of psychic boundary that I will elaborate here. I think that the use of the term *boundary violation* to describe sexual misconduct is damaging to our psychoanalytic profession because it minimizes the unique treatment that we provide and enacts elements of externalization of our responsibility as analysts.

When analysts have sex with patients, they are not operating within the basic contract and set of ideals that mark psychoanalytic work—that psychic boundaries will be discovered and understood through the analytic process. The concept of sexual boundary violation jumps from this psychical exploration and discovery of psychic boundary into inevitably moralistic and behavioral judgments. These judgments are intrinsic to maintaining ethical standards in the conduct of analytic work, but they do not involve the basic work approach to explore psychic boundaries at the heart of the analytic enterprise.

When Freud (1909) said that psychoanalysis is not an entirely "healthy" occupation, he was referring to the creation of illusion in psychoanalysis and the ritualized asymmetry of the procedure (see also Friedman, 2007). Freud (1915) elaborated that as analysts, we create illusion in order to help patients understand their desires, conflicts, and inhibitions. He was referring to the way in which the psychoanalytic setup helps to dissolve distinctions between conventional psychological domains, such as reality versus fantasy, in order to immerse both the patient and the analyst in processes that naturally lack distinction, or else function in relation to imaginary boundaries that are unconsciously constructed, sometimes in problematic ways. In this sense, psychoanalysis contributes to creating illusions in the service of working on disillusionment. But it is still rather unsavory to create illusions that will never be realized. The analytic task begins with this unsavory arrangement in the workplace. Anything good that will happen will be related to trying to work with the complex, frustrating, and gratifying play involving boundaries that are given up, lost, discovered, refound, hated, feared, loved, desired—boundaries that are obsolete but seemingly indispensable or desperately needed but missing.

I want to make a case for the notion that we reserve the term *boundary* for the psychic realm because the psychic boundaries of psychoanalysis are so fundamentally complex, dense, and intrinsically confusing that bringing in the realm of behavioral ethical violations is actually mystifying. We know that there is an invisible or barely visible boundary that divides everyday life from the particular frame of psychoanalytic work and that this boundary is crossed when analysts break from abstinence. Yet I believe that we already have and need to develop more precise ways to describe ethical violations involving analysts having sex with their patients than to describe them as boundary violations.

I will briefly explore some actual problems in using the term *boundary* in reference to both psychic and behavioral contexts. Some analysts writing about unethical conduct have also written about even psychic boundaries in ways that may add to our confusion. But I should make clear at the outset that in many ways, my wish to wrest the term *boundary* from its frequent companion, *violation,* and to separate psychic boundary from actual sexual behavior, is at least as much for aesthetic reasons as it is for technical clarity.

I suggest that there is an insidious way that our language about psychic boundaries has been juxtaposed in relation to sexual boundary violations. Paradoxically, I believe that the use of the term *boundary* to denote sexual misconduct involves a taming of the radical enterprise of psychoanalysis. The shift of the essential boundary concept from psychic to behavioral reflects not only the danger of sexual stimulation and intimacy in the analytic situation, but anxiety for all of us about loss of control in general in the analytic enterprise.

I believe that we enact a kind of disavowed claim for control over things that we do not control. So for example, aspects of relationships, analytic and otherwise, that we are all submerged in become analytic techniques, as if the analyst is now "using" these rather than submerged in them and trying to understand what is happening. I will provide an example of this confusion later in the paper when I discuss the problems inherent in thinking about patients' use of projective identification and identification as a "crossing of boundaries that we invite" (Gabbard, 2008).

Notes on the aesthetics of psychoanalysis as psychic boundary art

When Freud invented free association and the notion of the analyst allowing his mind to be adrift, he invented a new kind of art. He also invented a new kind of art when he essentially thematized subjectivity. Freud's invention of psychoanalysis, not unlike some other paradigm shifts in art, was a way of getting at another, different, and sometimes deeper subjectivity than that portrayed through our more conventional descriptions of the outside world.

Perhaps the most important issue related to boundaries that was understood by Freud is the automatic tendency for dissemblance. Our minds at once offer marvelous imaginative possibility and are to some extent prisons, representing constraint—boundaries that are sometimes unnecessary—that we have internalized and taken on board in becoming civilized. We seek escape. We are never entirely comfortable with the extent to which we are imprisoned, and as Nietzsche (1889) pointed out; our minds, through art, also provide us with opportunity for creative escape, solace, and excitement—"that without art we might die of boredom" (p. 79). Psychoanalysis, among other things, allows us to explore our discomfort and to help us determine if we can become more comfortable with constraints and to know more about our dissemblance in order that we may lead more creative lives.

Freud's invention put us permanently at risk of not knowing where his invention will take us. As Bromberg (2006, p. 135) has put it, psychoanalysts are "artists of uncertainty." Like Daedalus, the father of architecture who sought escape from imprisonment for he and his son Icarus, Freud invented analysis so that we might leave the bondage of internalized objects. Freud and Daedalus each invented methods that offer hope and opportunity for relief, but there is the possibility of pilot error, to be sure.

The art that Freud invented is what I think of as a kind of *boundary art*. The word *boundary* is itself a most complex word, given Freud's fundamental understanding of the unconscious as the driver of our own dissemblance and not knowing. I love the term *boundary* for its beauty, folly, and its ambitiously playful invitation to distort through illusions what we think we know that we don't really know. The term itself reflects the need we have as humans to earnestly, humorously, and sometimes pathetically locate where we are when we really don't know where we are. We put down stakes on a lonely and tiny frontier in a universe that is utterly indifferent to us, one that subjects each of us to an uncertain fate at an uncertain time. Boundaries help us to manage this overwhelming existential reality by creating illusions to facilitate speaking to each other about what we think we are saying that we cannot fully know we are saying.

Boundaries are shared illusions about what belongs to us and what belongs to the other. In psychoanalysis, we locate these blurring denotations with terms such as *fantasy, reality*, and *transference*. Boundaries are a part of how we play with our knowing and not knowing, our illusions, and our sadness about our limitations in knowing. Boundaries are pretend play words (omnipotent fantasies) about thinking that we own or are owned by a powerful other. The word itself allows us to think that we know the difference between self and other or the demarcation and coordinates between inside and outside. We are, in a sense, akin to small children saying that this is mine and that is yours through our use of the term *boundary.*

Boundary, in these senses of the word, involves as much verb as noun and is not unlike the word *play,* which while sometimes used as a noun is best understood as an activity. In fact, the concepts of boundary and play are really impossible to use without reference to the other. Play is always at work in psychoanalysis.

Central to my argument and to my understanding of psychoanalysis is that in beginning psychoanalysis, we are asking our patients to live outside the law in an unconventional terrain, one that loosens the rules of social and discursive engagement, in which we take liberties about translating what someone is saying that he doesn't know he is saying. That is license to kill. It is an artistic act to do this translating, this type of communicating. This living outside the law is what I mean by the analyst as a boundary artist, and it is why I regard what we do as a kind of therapeutic art. It is a kind of therapeutic art because it is explicitly described as a helping profession, something that most art is not. In fact, art may be among the most effective of the helping professions, but it is not usually explicitly described as such. To thematize subjectivity, another of Freud's primary inventions, is itself a therapeutic act, in all areas of human interaction.

In an essay entitled "The Wilderness of Childhood," Michael Chabon (2009) discussed a very disturbing shift in our very idea of childhood, in which adventure is no longer valued by our society in the way it once was. The wilderness of the outdoor life in suburbs is now occupied by neighbors, and for many children, scheduled activities have replaced unstructured time. In some ways, the adventures of saying what comes to mind are also minimized by our culture now. As Chabon wisely points out, one of the best ways to get to know a geographical place is to get lost in it a few times, really lost. I like this as an analogy to the notion of getting lost with our minds.

If, as David Foster Wallace (2009) once told an interviewer, the purpose of fiction is to give the reader, marooned in his own skull, access to the lives and minds of other selves, so the analytic patient associates, opens things up, and temporarily gets lost in order to gain access to other elements of his own selfhood. The abstract expressionist painter Richard Diebenkorn (1993) suggested that he seeks to "find an image that is more mine than the thought I had in my head" (p. 1).

As a boundary artist, the psychoanalyst maintains positions in various elements of psychic boundaries but is always aware of our tendency to become overly concrete in our ways of talking about boundaries. Since the particular border of everyday life and the rules of engagement in the framework of analysis are always a threat to be crossed in the imagination of the patient and analyst, and because they have been repeatedly crossed in the history and mythology of our everyday lives, it is easy for our imaginative capacities to become truncated. Repeated actual ethical transgressions and the threat of such may dull our connection to the technical craft required of the psychoanalyst as a boundary artist.

Among the most radical discoveries by Freud is that we really can't trust ourselves in knowing what we claim to know. There is more to us each than meets the eye. Our capacities for dissemblance make us unreliable knowers and narrators. The radical boundary problem in psychoanalytic work arises from the fact that we don't know all that we are saying and that we put our minds in the mind of a trained professional to see if he or she can help us understand or stand by more about what we were feeling or saying.

In a sense, psychoanalysis creates a new boundary, the frame which highlights what we don't know and what we think we know. I recall forty years ago when I began fly fishing, a guide had an interesting way of commenting to me as he watched my casts approaching a fish. He would assess whether it was worth continuing the floating fly approaching the trout. He would sometimes say, I like it, what do you think? If I agreed, he said, "let's let it float." This shared assessment about functional truth, functional possibility is constitutive of analytic space in which shared provisional understandings have their day. In psychoanalysis this is also quite complex because sometimes patients want us to know more than we know. The process of sharing uncertainty together is sometimes experienced as akin to sexual union, stimulation, or sexual exploration.

Contemporary analytic thinking that questions the authority of the analyst has done so partly because the unreliability of the analyst's mind is now better accepted as a given in the analytic situation. Bion had a great deal to do with advancing this particular idea, and of course it was developed significantly by the epistemological revolution in analytic thinking created by analysts such as Schafer, Mitchell, Donnel Stern, and Hoffman.

We are in a state of dissociated relationship to Shakespeare's dictum "This above all: To thine own self be true." We find ourselves in the midst of a confusion about the truth that we are trying to make sense of and to get some purchase on, always in some imperfect manner. Psychoanalysis is embedded in the notion that we seek some modicum of clarity about the nature of this dissociated relationship to the truth.

Boundary as activity involves our attempt to gain more purchase or clarity on our confusing relationship to our mind's truth. Inspiring analytic work, like very good written fiction or film, invites us to explore who is right and wrong—and yet, when all is said and done (never, by the way, is all said and done), ambiguity often reigns over clarity and harmony. Good analysis allows us to develop a greater capacity for holding this unsettling narrative. That is, in the end, what we do and what we help our patients to do.

There is a kind of complex mixture of earnestness and falseness to the analyst's request for the patient to take the leap of faith to say what comes to mind, another element of what makes analysis a not quite "healthy" line of work. As part of the method, the analyst wants the patient to free associate because he or she has been trained to understand what the patient is saying and has been analyzed in order to be useful to the patient without requiring the patient to gratify the analyst's own needs in too overpowering a manner.

The analyst, despite discomfort in making this request, nevertheless suggests it because it is part of the method (Cooper, 2010a, 2010b; Parsons, 2007). There is always a kind of false or counterphobic component to the invitation to say what comes to mind. Analysts, like our parents, do and do not want the patient to say everything that comes to mind and do and do not understand what's going on. They are, to varying degrees, anxious about how to be human beings and certainly about how to be analysts and parents. Some of us are more composed or confused about this than others. Some of us use defenses that minimize what we know, while others use defenses to buttress our illusions that we do know what's going on. But at some level, we are all in a state of existential, if not actual, equivalence about not knowing.

This element of dissemblance or inauthenticity on the part of the analyst is understandable and possibly unavoidable, but it is useful I think to remember that it is sometimes confusing to our patients. These types of dissemblance get worked out in good analyses as they are featured in transferences. Patients find the heart of the analyst, his strengths and weaknesses. Patients acclimate to our vulnerabilities, our forms of self-deception, our psychological limits. It is one of the hallmarks of working toward the depressive position that we feel our analyst's limitations in ways that are bearable, sometimes even helpful to us in bearing our own disappointments with others and self. When analysis gets more centrally organized around the limitations of the analyst, there is a much more serious impasse and stalemate.

The psychoanalyst as a boundary artist works at the border of the concrete and symbolic, figurative and abstract, in the borderlands of fantasy and consensual reality, dream and waking life. This borderland is where we live in figuring out what comes from the patient's mind, our own mind, and the third psychic realities that emerge from patient and analyst being together. Our language in psychoanalysis is the border language of metaphor. We are engaged in collaborative art with our patients. Nietzsche's notion of art as involving the transformation of reality into something creative and less boring describes a great deal of what we do in analysis by trying to make the familiar unfamiliar in order to gain purchase on it. Through the use of metaphor as our border language, we are trying to see something new about what is apparent, in a sense questioning what is obvious as a defensive construction.

In a certain way, relative to conventional discourse and our other non-familial relationships, psychoanalysis begins with the frightening fact that we are trying to enter into the patient's mind. Bolognini (2010, p. 32) interestingly described psychoanalysis as a form of "psychic cohabitation". Levin (2014) suggested that it might also be considered as a kind of "mutual mental squatting." For after all, as analysis develops, patients learn that they have entered into our minds.

I find it especially useful to think about analysis as beginning with the two participants entering and living in the minds of the other. This view stands in contrast to the way that we think about these processes as exclusively developing through transference. While transference involves the deepening of these experiences about how we live in each other's minds, in certain ways, the concept of transference also introduces a distinction that allows us to get more distance on this boundary blurring. Freud's (1915) original observations about transference focused on transference as the patient's way of including the analyst in his neurosis. In other words, transference is not only what makes our relationship to one another more blurry. It is also what provides figurability and understanding about how we live in the minds of each other.

Freud discovered that transference is a universal psychic phenomenon of the human mind and that this tendency is embedded in social discourse. He also noticed that the therapeutic relationship is nearly coterminous with what has been called the psychotherapeutic setting (Modell, 1991). This realization, among his most important and vexing contributions to the theory of technique, established that the boundary between what comes from the patient and analyst would be blurred. But he also insisted that the power of the method rests on the capacity to *maintain* this level of complexity and blurring.

Parsons (2006) expresses beautifully the need for the analyst to maintain an openness to the blurring of psychic boundaries in stating that

> The most important happenings in both the analyst's and the patient's internal worlds lie at the boundary between conscious and unconscious, and the nature of an analyst's interventions depends on how fully what happens at that boundary is articulated in the analyst's consciousness.
>
> (p. 1193)

Parat (1976) as well as anyone makes the case for the notion that analysts are boundary artists, in that our best interventions in some sense short circuit consciousness. And of course Keats's (1952) notion of negative capability got at the same phenomena: to be "capable of being in uncertainties, Mysteries, doubts, without any irritable reaching after fact and reason" (p. 37).

It is simultaneously obvious but in some ways unseen how psychoanalysis itself contains elements of boundary confusion and boundary crossing in terms of what we don't know that we are trying to know. Psychoanalysis is predicated on the exploration of the patient's mind as experienced and translated through the analyst's mind, with all of its strengths and vulnerabilities. Indeed, psychoanalysis explores the terrain between what is inside and what is outside, what is old and new, and what is clear but later seen as defensively clear because it gave us a signpost for a period of time. I am reminded of a refrain from a Leonard Cohen song, "tonight will be fine, will be fine … for a while." Psychoanalysis explores what is known to us and what lies in the vast territory of the psychic unknown.

The artistry of psychoanalysis is to transform psychic pain into something that is more bearable or, in the best of circumstances, even something that we might use to live more creatively. As Rilke (1922) put it, "Beauty is nothing but the beginning of terror that we are still just able to bear" (p. 35). As analysts we try to develop this capacity to bear terror and ugliness. Clive Bell (1914) stated that "The artist is not trying to produce pretty or even beautiful form, he is engaged in the most important task of re-creating his ruined internal world and the resulting form will depend on how well he succeeds in his task" (p. 59). The patient is a creator and onlooker to this beauty and ruin, and as analysts, we are trying to help bear and hold this ruined state.

Caution is well-advised, but too much caution means that we might never make contact with the patient and thus not help the patient to make contact with new parts of himself. Too little caution means that we might overwhelm the patient and actually make him feel his "catastrophe" (Bion, 1959, p. 101) more vividly and without hope for integration. Perhaps this position is related to one described by Richard Diebenkorn (1993) in his "Notes to Myself on Beginning a Painting." He stated that he aims "to be careful only in a perverse way" (p. 1). As it relates to the analytic situation, and particularly the question of boundaries, being careful in a perverse way involves the analyst's self-reflective adventurousness in trying to know about the patient's and his own related wilderness. We are perverse in knowing that we cannot undo the catastrophe of what Bion (1959) described as the missing function. Our efforts are perversely guided by the awareness that we offer a different kind of help than the patient might desire. But we are careful in that we do this as translators and readers of what patients may be communicating they didn't know they wanted to convey.

For me, ideally, the framework of psychoanalysis is nearly always offered with carefulness in a perverse way. This is embodied in the adventurousness and unconventional nature of saying what comes to mind in the context of a treatment. The late historian Tony Judt (2010) defined the edge and "edge people" as "the place where countries, communities, allegiances, affinities, and roots bump uncomfortably up against one another—where cosmopolitanism is not so much an identity as the normal condition of life" (p.2). The analyst as a boundary artist is helping people to live on the edge of their own internal cosmopolitanism, and there is no doubt that the capacity to live in this place with another person is a privilege for both patient and analyst.

As Parsons (2007) has put it: "we need to be aware of our disturbance by the process and the patient needs to feel our emotional availability" (p. 1194). Getting lost in the wilderness at times is required.

Another conceptual boundary related to the psychic concept of boundary

I am concerned that the terminological use of boundary in the context of sexual misconduct is part of a particular kind of distortion of what we do and do not have control of in relation to psychic mechanisms and psychic functioning. Aesthetics come into play because in my view, the concept of psychic boundary involves the workable artistic function of the analyst as a boundary artist. The use of the term boundary to refer to analysts who engage in sexual misconduct in some sense involves the unwitting taming of the radical and artistic notion of psychic boundary. Use of the term boundary to describe unethical behavioral referents, usually coupled with violation, degrades it by forcing retreat from the complexity of the kinds of psychic boundary that I have been describing. In fact, among the most radical of Freud's and Klein's discoveries is that in thinking about the concept of boundary, we have to begin with the notion that we are speaking in large part about boundary as a fantasy. I think that we have enough to parse related to psychic boundaries without extending the term to cover behavioral misconduct. It is our job to psychologically understand these violations as we are trained to do, but in order to do this part of our work well, we need to avoid the confusion that arises from hijacking the lynchpin concept in psychoanalysis—boundary—to provide a global and vague reference point for this behavior.

One could reasonably argue that my developing attempt here to create some distinct lines between psychical boundaries and sexual misconduct is also illusory. I believe that the clear and distinct line between psychical boundaries and sexual misconduct could be thought of as a fiction constitutive of the analytic space in our particular culture. I am more comfortable with that fiction than one that speaks more globally of sexual misconduct as boundary violation.

The conceptualization of sexual misconduct and actual behavior in terms of boundaries gives rise to another different kind of problem when the same term also plays an essential role in describing the many psychic borders that patients and analysts traverse in the course of analytic work.

I want to say in advance that I am going to take on what at first glance appears to be a very small matter about the way we use language, and I'm going to amplify it for discursive purposes. I will focus on some particular words from my colleague Glen Gabbard, who has been at the forefront of exploring what he refers to as the analyst's ethical boundary violations. I do so in order to provide a critique of this usage. I do not mean to minimize his significant contributions to understanding unethical behavior among our colleagues. I suspect that he might agree with the point I want to make, but our words matter, particularly since the notion of psychic boundaries is so central to the art of psychoanalysis.

In many discussions of boundaries in psychoanalysis, the word is referred to in terms of ethical and sexual boundary breaking—boundary violations as a behavioral action (e.g., Gabbard & Lester,

1995). Analysts also refer to boundaries as including psychical structural characteristics of the analytic relationship that refer to frame, emphasizing experiences of safety for the patient that I want to preserve. But in using the term in both psychic and behavioral contexts, we conflate those matters in analytic work that we aim to have control over (e.g., the analyst's abstinence and behavioral conduct) and psychical dimensions of the analytic setting that we have no control over, such as the patient's unconscious slips of the tongue, telling of dreams, and the use of projective identification.

For example, consider a comment made by Gabbard (2008) in a discussion of a paper by Goldberg (2008) dealing with boundaries. Gabbard (2008) makes the following intriguing statement: "Paradoxically, the boundaries that we set up in the analytic setting are established so that both participants have the possibility of crossing them psychologically." He provides as examples of boundary crossing: "familiar modes of crossing the semipermeable membrane constructed by the analytic dyad, introjection, projective identification and empathy" (p.878).

I believe that Gabbard is trying here to distinguish between the use of *boundary* as related to behavior versus uses of the term *psychic boundary* that relate to unconscious mechanisms and fantasy. Psychic boundaries relate to the intrinsic confusion of human communication about what is inside and outside and what is self and other. He is referring to the basic concept of abstinence as what allows us to do our work, an unassailably logical argument and, in my view, an absolute prerequisite to analytic work.

Yet there is something that is subtly quite provocative about Gabbard's understanding of the analyst's power in his description here. I think that I know what he might intend to mean when he says that abstinence is what "allows" the patient and analyst to "cross boundaries psychologically." I believe that what he means to say is that we have the possibility of understanding these psychic processes with the patient in analytic work. But what does the phrase mean— that we create a rule of abstinence so that each participant is allowed to cross psychic boundaries expressed through unconscious mechanisms of projective identification, identification, and empathy?

It is likely that Gabbard's intention is to suggest that the creation of the frame itself (that kind of boundary) allows us to notice, explore, and make use of understanding the processes of projective identification and empathy. But I focus on the way that he puts it because it expresses a problem that we as psychoanalysts continually enact related to the borders of what we do and do not control in the analytic arrangement. I don't conceptualize the boundary of abstinence established by analysts in the analytic setting so that we can cross boundaries of projective identification, empathy, or identification in the analytic setting because I don't consider psychic phenomena such as empathy, projective identification, or enactment as forms of boundary crossing. There are only boundaries in the fantasies and affective life of those who listen to the psychic adventures of the other. Being clear about that is helpful to patients and to us professionally with each other. In psychoanalysis, the concept of boundary is always considered in the context of fantasies about boundaries.

The only way to understand projective identification or identification as a boundary crossing, it seems to me, is if we think about the differentiation of self and other in ways that involve sharp distinctions within the intersubjective field. Actually these sharp distinctions really have no place in a field theory of human communication. I believe that much of the professional use of the term "boundary violation" in connection with sexual misconduct is based on some of these quite concrete definitions of self and other that minimize the ways that projective identification is a part of everyday life. Just as Freud discovered transference as a function of the human mind (even if it is more conspicuous in the analytic setting), so did Klein discover projective identification as a form of human communication. And as many have pointed out, it is partly the basis of empathy as well (e.g. Ogden, 1979).

I would say, alternatively, that projective identification exists as a need that humans have "as deep as hunger and thirst" (Ogden, 2004, p. 173). Psychoanalysts set up rules about abstinence in the analytic situation to provide real and illusory experiences of safety, ideals held by professional organizations that the analyst belongs to about the invasive procedure of psychoanalysis. These rules allow us to look at psychological processes that are not really acknowledged in conventional discourse. Psychoanalysts simply construct a situation that allows us to understand the embedded complexity of psychic boundaries. Empathy and projective identification occur naturalistically unless we begin with a notion that self and other are so clearly differentiated from the get-go.

Conventional discourse enacts the processes of projective identification, empathy, and identification. Humor is funny because we are putting things into the other person that are fundamentally uncontainable related to aggression, hypocrisy, longings, repulsion, shame, rage, and so on. Projective identification and empathy, transference and countertransference are not reflections of our invitation for boundary crossing in psychoanalysis. Instead, they reflect the ways in which minds communicate in intersubjective patterns that in psychoanalysis we try to fleetingly understand. These processes of human communication are generally not really acknowledged in conventional discourse, yet they are the foundational principles upon which psychoanalysis works. For we can't understand what people are telling us that they don't know they are telling us without our empathic capacities and attunement to projective identification. What we do invite is an opportunity for patients to talk about whatever comes to mind, to psychically shed their clothes, and to discuss things that we are taught from childhood not to discuss with others. These processes are not something that the analyst is involved in offering, controlling, or approving. Instead, these processes are embedded in human communication. We do not approve them. We use them.

These messages to our patients about heightened expressiveness in the context of behavioral restraint are, as Modell (1991) has described, paradoxical in nature, and abstinence helps therapists to *cope* with implicit paradox in the structural arrangements of psychoanalysis. Paradox exists between the rule of abstinence in the framework of treatment and another boundary between everyday life in which abstinence is not required, even if sometimes advised depending on the social context. Describing our needs to cope with paradoxical and impossibly complex elements of the analytic situation that we don't create allows for a clearer statement about the relationship between abstinence and psychic communication that we have no control over. As I said earlier, I imagine that Gabbard would agree with this formulation, but I draw attention to these words because these ways of thinking permeate all of our analytic thinking and may enact ways that we try to control matters we have no control over in the context of our impossible profession.

Why did we ever go in the direction of referring to engaging in sex with patients as a boundary violation? I actually see it as a form of abstraction and defense on the part of the analytic community— a shying away from the very specific ways that we are uniquely qualified to elaborate. We do so in describing the pathology and regressive elements of our patients, but in describing our colleagues, who deserve our compassion, we offer obfuscation and abstraction. By referring to unethical sexual conduct as a boundary violation, are we again unconsciously trying to bring unethical behavior into some element of our technical setup related to the psychic use of boundaries? I have a hunch that we are.

By characterizing psychic phenomena as involving boundaries that we invite patients to cross, such as projective identification, we are potentially involved in a particular kind of professional enact-ment—the conscription of naturalistically occurring human commu-nication patterns into the service of the analyst's sense of control and dominance. In other words, we enact a kind of disavowed claim for control over things that we do not control. So for example, aspects of relationships, analytic and otherwise, that we all employ become analytic techniques, as if the analyst is now "using" these rather than submerged in them and trying to understand what is happening. That both people are submerged in the process is not to say that there is absolute mutuality or symmetry; I think that there is a great deal of asymmetry in our roles, and presumably the ana-lyst is in a better position than the patient to make sense of what is happening.

I suspect that these problems are even more pronounced when sexual misconduct is involved in the discussion of boundary cross-ing. I think that it is safe to say that analysts, like all human beings, are frightened and anxious about their own sexuality and others'. It is not by accident that this unjustified conscription of technique about psychical boundaries to the power and authority of the ana-lyst is made by many of us, because I believe that it unconsciously works to titrate the analyst's anxiety about an area that, along with death, is the most anxiety-producing area of work in psychoanalysis. It seems to me that to be open to our patients' sexualities and all elements of projective identification, including anger and wishes for merger, involves a recognition that we often, if not always, ask our patients to submit to our own comfort levels and thresholds for listening to affect and fantasy. We are bound to accept this more directly than to create a construction of technique in which we make inaccurate claims about what we allow and don't allow.

Each of us as analyst is required to know what we allow and don't allow as it relates to behavior. We also know that we are engaged in a similar conscious and unconscious communication to our patients about what we can tolerate regarding sexual desire and hostility. I have been aware of how I've conveyed my own limits to patients with very strong erotic interests or strong angry feelings.

We are all guilty of the conscription or sliding of elements of communication, such as projective identification, into a technical framework (e.g., referring to it as a matter of technique) that we call psychoanalysis. In other words, we are all subject to developing descriptions of technique that involve subtle shifts to safety in the service of control and reduction of anxiety.

We all fear the wilderness.

Note

1 A different version of this paper was previously published in Steven Cooper, *The analyst's experience of the depressive position,* New York & London: Routledge, 2016. The author greatly appreciates the editorial generosity, sharpening of ideas and general clarity provided by Charles Levin.

References

Bell, C. (1914). *Art.* London: Frederick A. Stokes Company Publishers.

Bion. (1959). Attacks on linking. In *Second thoughts* (pp. 93–109). London: Karnac, 1984.

Bolognini, S. (2010). *Secret passages: The theory and technique of inter psychic relations.* New York & London: Routledge (New Library of Psychoanalysis).

Bromberg, P. M. (2006). *Awakening the dreamer.* Hillsdale: The Analytic Press.

Celenza, A., & Gabbard, G. O. (2003). Analysts who commit sexual boundary violations: A lost cause? *Journal of the American Psychoanalytic Association, 51,* 617–636.

Chabon, M. (2009, July 16). Manhood for amateurs: The wilderness of childhood. *New York Review of Books, 56* (12), 11–14.

Cooper, S. (2010a). Self-criticism and unconscious grandiosity: Transference-countertransference dimension. *International Journal of Psychoanalysis, 91*, 1115–1136.

Cooper, S. (2010b). *A disturbance in the field: Essays in transference-countertransference.* New York: Routledge.

Diebenkorn, R. (1993). Notes to myself on beginning a painting. Unpublished notes.

Freud, S. (1909). Letter to Jung, Letter 134F. In W. McGuire (Ed.), *The Freud-Jung letters: The correspondence between Sigmund Freud and C. G. Jung* (pp. 209–211). Cambridge, MA: Harvard University Press, 1974.

Freud, S. (1915). Observations on transference-love. In J. Strachey (Ed. & Trans.), *The standard edition of the complete psychological works of Sigmund Freud* (Vol. 12, pp. 157–173). London, UK: Hogarth Press.

Friedman, L. (2007). The delicate balance of work and illusion in psychoanalytic. *Psychoanalytic Quarterly, 76*, 817–833.

Gabbard, G. O. (1994). Sexual excitement and countertransference love in the analyst. *Journal of the American Psychoanalytic Association, 42*, 1083–1106.

Gabbard, G. O. (2008). Boundaries, technique, and self-deception: A discussion of Arnold Goldberg's "Some limits of the boundary concept". *Psychoanalytic Quarterly, 77*, 877–881.

Gabbard, G. O., & Lester, E. P. (1995). *Boundaries and boundary violations in psychoanalysis.* New York: Basic Books.

Goldberg, A. (2008). Some limits of the boundary concept. *Psychoanalytic Quarterly, 77*, 861–875.

Judt, T. (2010). Edge people. *New York Review of Books, pages 1-3.* February 23, 2010.

Keats, J. (1952). *Letters* (4th ed.) (M. B. Forman, Ed.). London: Oxford University Press.

Levin, C. (2014). Personal communication.

Modell, A. H. (1991). The therapeutic relationship as paradoxical experience. *Psychoanalytic Dialogues, 1*, 13–28.

Nietzsche, F. (1889). *Twilight of the idols.* New York: Hackett Publishing Company.

Ogden, T. (1979). On projective identificaton. *International Journal of Psycho-Analysis, 60*, 357–373.

Ogden, T. (2004). The analytic third: Implications for psychoanalytic theory and technique. *Psychoanalytic Quarterly, 73*, 167–196.

Parat, C. J. (1976). À propos du contre-transfert [On countertransference]. *Revue Française de Psychanalyse, 40*, 545–560.

Parsons, M. (2006). The analyst's countertransference to the psychoanalytic process. *International Journal of Psychoanalysis, 87*, 1183–1198.

Parsons, M. (2007). Raiding the inarticulate: The internal analytic setting and listening beyond countertransference. *International Journal of Psychoanalysis*, *88*, 1441–1456.

Rilke, R. (1922). *Duino elegies*. New York: Caranet Press.

Wallace, D. (2009). *Book tour comments*. Cambridge, MA.

Winnicott, D.W. (1971). *Playing and Reality*. Harmondsworth, Middlesex: Penguin.

Chapter 8

When the body knows the mind's rest[1]

Stephen Hartman

The location of desire: the field and the rest

When Muriel Dimen's generative paper, *Lapsus Linguae or a Slip of the Tongue* was posted online, it became a focal point for conversation about sexual boundary violations (IARPP Colloquium, May 2011). *Lapsus Linguae* quickly put a human face on an erstwhile stone-faced (if not poker-faced) problem. As a result of Dimen's brave self-disclosure, it became possible to locate the mind and body of the analyst as a professional in a multi-dimensional, embodied field rife with projected identification, dissociation, and power. So very articulate in this regard, Dimen made it clear that these collective dynamics are inherent to clinical work. Any future inquiry into sexual boundary violations will have to contend with her unique way of plotting disciplinary structures and psychological structures in psychic space and physical space to depict a psychosocial nexus where boundary violation happens. (See also Dimen, 2000, 2011b, 2014).

Lapsus Linguae is also a text about silence. Insofar as it is a tale of tongues—tied and then untied, it concerns language and bodies as well as motion and emotion. And insofar as Muriel asks us to pause and reflect viscerally on aspects of psychic reality that simmer in the erotized space between analyst and patient before coming to boil in a boundary violation, it is a text about the relationship between space, sexuality, and their ungainly representation in "mindfulness." To call this space "erotic transference," "the sensory floor" (Goldberg, 2012), the Interpersonal Relational Field (Stern, 2013), "the setting" (Green, 1975), or the *emergent* Bionian *field* (Baranger and Baranger, 2008;

Ferro, 2009; Peltz and Goldberg, 2013) would be to diminish Dimen's contribution which moves beyond the *mind* loading of these "field" theories to deal with what I will call *the rest*. Indeed, *the rest* conjures a minefield prior to symbolization and, even in its unrepresented form, it carries more affect than a phenomenological communication yet utters less meaning than can be linked to in a mind-field. It is a not yet embodied, not yet conscious, not yet symbolized movement among, toward, and away from desire.

If not mind exactly, *the rest* that Dimen identifies is not the province of the body either, nor sexuality in its discursive form (Foucault, 1977). Yes, this mind/body synapse resists Cartesian representation, but it is neither the fallout from the collapse of body impinging on mind nor a kind of heterotopic "other space" (Foucault, 1986) where a rhizomatic antidote to binary structures of power/knowledge takes shape (Deleuze and Guattari, 1977, 1987, Foucault, 1980). Rather, kin to Laplanche's *le sexuel* (Laplanche, 2003/2011; Stein, 2007), it resembles the embodied fumes of historical, psychic-social and cultural excess that flood the self in what Winnicott (1988) called the psyche-soma.[2] Call it a "relational primitive State" if you like, but it is not yet a state unto itself. As a space where a sense of self comes to *rest* (rather than reside—because its tenure is precarious), it is something more like an intervention in the anthropological "field" as described by Clifford Geertz (1973).

Geertz noted how the effort to document an emergent event in the field inevitably changed it according to the rules that the anthropologist imported into the field to describe it. "Culture is public," he wrote, "because meaning is" (1973, p. 12). From this perspective, neither the anthropologist nor the analyst is in a position to understand what is going on in the "field" because of the field's liminal correspondence to each participant's version of "reality." The analyst is more in the position of accidental meaning-maker than of lucid understander, and this underlying condition of the relationship always places the patient's meaning in jeopardy. The analyst's footprint in the interpersonal field is like the sound of a falling tree in the "forest of symbols" (Baudelaire, 1954; Turner, 1967): it may only be heard by chance; its coercive existence may go unnoticed and so, too, its symbolic heft *in a deep and tenebrous unity*.

If the field in mainstream psychoanalysis is an extension of Freud's intrapsychic dream theory (Ferro, 2009), one that trolls for and consolidates meanings, Dimen's field decenters and multiplies the sources of field effects and "correspondences."[3] Her cultural field is one that speaks to us in tongues—where the analyst is always already at risk of becoming the spokesperson for *the rest*—the helpful church minister or sage rabbi who urges us to let bygones be bygones.

I'm using the term "the rest" in a number of confounding yet overlapping ways to demonstrate how densely saturated the psycho-social field is in excess bodily meaning. "The rest" signifies any number of cultural conditions, social configurations, psychic hurdles, and internal objects that one must always manage when confronted, as Schilder (1950) put it, with "the image and appearance of the human body." Our "body schema" is never isolated. It has the constant task of representing more than it can physically see or touch. Body images "are always encircled by the body images of others" (1950, p. 240); consequently, "erotic exchanges in the body-image are always social phenomena and are accompanied by the corresponding phenomena in the body-images of others."

The rest is a murky overlap of factors, Schilder explains: "there is a continuous interchange between parts of our own body-image and the body-images of others. There is projection and apersonization. But in addition the whole body-image of others is taken in (identification) or our own body-image can be pushed out as a whole" (p. 241).[4] *The body's rest*, as I am using the term, is never static: "there is not only the continual change in our own body-image but also the continual changes in its spatial relations, emotional relations of the body-images of others and the construction of the body-images of others" (p. 241). And all this prior to representation.

The rest is at once the extra that can be consciously accounted for and the excess that is enigmatically not-quite represented in the unconscious (Laplanche, 1999; Scarfone, 2015). It is the rest of "them" and at the same time the not/me in me. Even in repose, there is the rest. *To rest* can mean "take a break," "stay put," "be assured of," "relax," or "retreat" (among other actions) given the registration of bodies and minds leaning on or impinging upon one another. There is no rest without *the* rest and yet *the rest*, as I see it, is often little more than a quiver in the inter-psyche-soma. As meaning, it is public because power is. As unformulated meaning it is at once the jury and the choir, the echo and the ghost, the finger and the ring, depending on the liminality of the subject vis à vis the rest (McGleughlin, 2015a, 2015b). And so the rest is always already the audience (Levin, 2015) to movement that has and hasn't yet happened: the un-born gesture in disorganized attachment (Asibong, 2015), the yet-to-happen in panic, and the ah-ha! in *nachträglichkeit*.

Once noticed, the emergent rest cannot be deduced from an encapsulated field as if a byproduct of impasses and enactments or the progeny of containment. It is not yet so stable—and certainly not as codified as the theoretical constructs we use to wrest the rest: an arrest such as psychoanalysis has accomplished with the "primal scene." It is the liminal space *between* that Dimen has been mapping in her work for many years: *desire in the space of difference* (Dimen, 1991; Dimen and Goldner, 2002), a hybrid space *between lust and libido* (1999) that yields, recalling Bhabha (1994, p. 15), the location of desire as an antidote to "the forgetting of the unhomely moment." Dimen locates slips of the tongue in Foucault's (1977) manner of describing "resistances" which is a move beyond Ferenczi's (1949) confusion of tongues. It is not a repressed memory or dissociated cognition that surfaces in the location of desire, but the invocation of repression as viewed from a liminal position toward normative desire (Guralnik, 2011; McGleughlin, 2015b).

What makes Dimen's field work so profound is precisely that it concerns the collapse of the in-between space wherein boundaries are violated in recursive relation to the location wherein they become vested. Peltz and Goldberg (2013) recently commented that Stern's (2013) comparisons of the relational and Bionian approaches to "the field" were describing two very distinct entities: the former descriptive of *relating* and the latter a portrait of *encounter*. Without rehearsing their argument in detail here, I wish simply to argue that Dimen resolves the binary between relating and encounter by placing these "constituent aspects of the field" in a preponderant recursive relationship. Relating creates encounter, which in turn creates relating, which in turn creates encounter, and on and on until there is neither relating nor encounter. This is the charged condition under which a "boundary violation" may develop—one potent enough to locate the mind in the body's rest.

The reader will understand from this last statement that in this chapter I am deliberately trying to destabilize the over-determined sense of our disciplinary jargon, in particular the phrase "boundary violation." I shall be arguing that the ethical quandary of psycho-analysis revolves around its instantiation of a transitional or potential space in which it becomes possible for a constitutive boundary viola-tion to occur—one that relocates the mind in terms of the rest—that is, in relation to everything that has been left over and out in the pro-cess of "emotional development."[5] This transformational potential of the analytic situation can be powerful and seductive; it may engender in either patient or analyst an overvaluation of the analyst's command of the "field," setting the stage for the psychic tragedy of a boundary *mis*-violation.

Without splitting the body and the mind into a binary, pitting the analytic dyad into complementary roles of splitter and container, or extracting individual dynamics from the collective history of inter-loping bodies and desires, Dimen expresses a very clear insight about human nature: desire must find a place in the mind—which requires it to find a place in the Other's mind—so that it can rest in the body. This process is necessarily *restless* because of the uneven-ness of power deemed culturally and professionally necessary to the binaries (e.g. ego/id, Freud, 1923/1961; container/contained; Bion, 1962; mutual/asymmetrical; Hoffman, 1983) that are theorized to explicate subjectivity and are thus encoded in the clinical practices that "demonstrate" *it*.

Returning to boundary violations, then, let's note that Ferenczi's experiments in mutual analysis have been described as the effort to frustrate binary positions rather than the analysand so that one might describe intersubjective psychic space (Carnochan, 2001). Bion's (1962) demand that the analyst eschew memory and desire portions out the frame so that an analytic encounter may give voice to the mind's pre-established links. Dimen's recursive approach to field work does not cordon-off the traumatic violation so that inter-subjective meaning might be made. As with Salamon's (2010) "felt sense of the body," Dimen recognizes a necessary tension among psychosocial and material boundaries. She takes Ferenczi and Bion a step further into the social domain, where subjectivity percolates in the *always already* that brought the dyad together in the first place. Then she looks back at what had seemed obvious about the scene of care to warn us how readily the dislocation of boundaries that foster intersubjective and inter-embodied knowing of psychic space is frustrated by exploitation within the frame and dissolved into silence.

When one must talk about what the body knows when the mind (or minds) cannot yet represent, a *lapsus linguae*, a muteness, about the body prevails almost as a kind of protest (Gerson, 2011) but more experientially as submission (Benjamin, 1988; Ghent, 1990). Coupled with sex panic, weighed in afterward time, a lapse in representation frames a hectic yet stalled moment when bodies register mind's necessary erotic restlessness. In this lapse between time and representation, between the enigmatic message and the disembodied vocoder of the dissociated soul, inter-embodied boundary work transpires.

In celebration of Dimen's foray into turf that at once eew's and ah's (Dimen, 2005), I will discuss nonverbal moments when tongues probe the location of desire in what Winnicott (1988) called the "psyche-soma." These are itinerant moments of eros that convene in the boundary between self and Other so as to facilitate a connection between one's mind and one's body that allows desire a home. Dimen demonstrates how unnamed urges flow among bodies in ways that allow a person to locate desire in a body and a mind of her own and, in turn, to develop an embodied mindfulness of Others that grounds a sense of ethical responsibility in the body— one that, on discovery, seems to have been always already there albeit trumped by the obviousness of power (Althusser, 1971).

After Winnicott (1988), I am concerned with the subject's location of desire in and between bodies in a "psycho-somatic field." I take Winnicott's observation that "the mind is a specialized part of the psyche that is not necessarily body-linked" (p. 53) to imply that one discovers desire in the same environmental/social conditions that give rise to a sense of self. This quest to locate desire is "temporal" with the objective of having one's own desire and "procedural" as a project of knowing it (recall Ogden's (2004) synthesis of holding and containing). When the psyche-soma locates the mind in the body in this recursive manner, desire becomes *useful* to the self. By contrast to Kristeva's (1995) notion that the psyche's operations on language notate the soul within the psyche-soma, I argue that there is a charged boundary between self and other, a psychic space where the body knows the minds' rest in anticipation of boundary's collapse. By this I mean that the various permeabilities of bodies and minds in this space, under conditions that foster reflection—what Winnicott called "quiet" —can be accommodated within a sensation that we know as *desire*. Within desire, objects are (and were) in motion before we have object representations and after they return from the no-man's land of orgasm (Rundel, 2015; Sake-ketopoulou, 2014). Desiring begets the soul. Often and necessarily, this nonverbal space is recognized because it is violated.

Boundary violations of a generative sort link an instinctive need to locate desire in our person (or psyche-soma) in the presence of another person. At the same time, the successful negotiation of this violation links us to the social prehistory of mind—just as it links our emergent *souls* to the humanness of the body—but in a manner that is not easily represented to mind. A violation of this boundary that is ethical acknowledges the relational matrices that endow the psyche. A perverse violation of this boundary twists the tongue in restless (k)nots.

Violations: necessary and perverse

It's my great fortune to have a polyglot relationship with Muriel Dimen. After twenty years of dialogue, first as a graduate student, then analytic candidate, supervisee, mentee, neighbor, co-teacher, co-editor, general accomplice and, most recently, discussant of her work, I cherish the sound of her many voices. Not long ago, after a long day of presenting in a seminar, I sensed in her a muted voice. I've heard it before—after a brainy spree at a conference or board meeting, a kind of uncomfortably numb feeling. Muriel is not one to relish numbing out: always at the ready especially when her reserves are low. I think this occasion was the first time—after a complex presentation with a large and inscrutable group—that Muriel and I walked together in silence. I knew that her gait was articulating her mind's need for rest. I tried to pace her as we ambled, uneasy at first. I found our nonverbal numbness unnerving since I've always looked to Dimen's stride to affirm my own.

It's an honor to have the experience of collateral solitude. When Winnicott (1958) described being alone in the presence of an Other, he must have intended the conceptual leap from maternal embrace to a moment like this, a moment when communication between two quiet bodies knows the mind's un-rest yet leaves it be. One is left alone *enough* for stimulating "dreams" and self-referential worries to cohere as tolerable qualities of being human. One is thus connected to and held by Others in a natural history of minds and bodies that unites us to the collective beyond our selves (Doi, 1989; Gonzalez, 2012).

Neither Muriel nor I endure an unquiet interpersonal field without hyper-gymnastic introspection. That day, stumbling along, it was simply evident that one ought not address the un-quiet of our walk so that a boundary that had already been crossed in the psyche-soma might be respected in the *reality* of persons. Above all else, Winnicott (1988, p. 103) appreciated how necessary "a delicate initiation of a relationship" is during such restless moments in the psyche-soma. He explained: "integration feels sane" when a restless mind is allowed to "feel mad to be losing integration that has been acquired" (1988, p. 118) in the presence of an Other whose soma recognizes (can identify with or at least imagine) the others' mind's unrest. One may then locate a personal mind in a sense of one's own body moving among Others with concern and gratitude. After a few blocks in silence, Muriel and I found a rhythm and it was a relief to just be tired and a bit mute, peripatetic bodies with quiet minds.

It is not a relief to know that Dimen's voice was so-long muted as the result of a sexual boundary *mis*-violation by her first analyst. Her elegant paper, *Lapsus Linguae* (Laplanche, 2003/2011) and the publications that followed from it are written in her most eloquent voice to date. Ironically, the paper traces a subtle history of muteness in Dimen's powerful dialect. Suddenly, certain tambours that edge below sensation on the decibel scale are audible. Had we heard them all along? Did we hear them somehow but not know it? Did she? Did her analyst? Did we or did he respond, contain, ignore, violate something in the psyche/soma surround that left a mark on the Richter Scale only after Muriel (then analysand, now a training analyst) told us the rest of the *unspeakable* story?

It was the *unrest* of the story that she told us, really. Dimen's uncharacteristic silence references the disciplinary action of *the Real* when the un-real colonized her body and mind. If the reality of one's need to become mindful of desire is fostered in a secure holding environment, the boundary between self and other is represented in what Winniott named transitional space. The boundary is mutable through the accumulative gestures of two subjects at play. Muteness portrays mind's dislocation in a disturbance of the boundary between self and other. In a clash between the Law, the body, and the psyche, the mind cannot locate itself in the body to which it belongs (Guralnik and Simeon, 2010; Hartman, 2010). Unrest endures in depersonalized and mute self-states because the necessary crossing of excitement and quiet goes internal—and reality becomes a matter of circumnavigating boundaries rather than surrendering to their usefulness (Ghent, 1990, 1992). This is how I would define *mis-violation*.

Just as failures in parenting are generative of the illusions that foster creativity (Winnicott, 1951), I have argued that violations of reality are often necessary so that an unquiet mind can be located in a body that has an alien dream (Hartman, 2013a).[6] When this developmental need to reconcile what Winnicott (1988, p. 100) called "quiet and excited relationships" with external reality cannot be represented without dangerous recourse, it is a perverse violation. Perverse violations disavow *the Law's* grip on the spatialization of mind according to the logic that structures authority. Here, in afterward time, we see how Foucault's (1979) *panopticon*, a prison that needs no guards because the prisoners have been induced to patrol themselves, becomes a function of perverse boundary violations.

When a trusted male authority vested by our profession with confidence and judgment abuses that trust and remains silent, confident that he need never speak about his lapse in judgment, a perverse boundary violation in the treatment is supported by the structural logic that professional asymmetry is necessary to quality care. The patient is left with two choices: join the analyst in a perverse disavowal of reality (Dor, 1999; Stein, 2005) or occupy a place of unrest. Each position comes at great cost to the capacity to locate one's mind in one's body and, therefore, one's desire in a matrix of ethical concern.

The third option is to speak. But this places the analysand at risk in the presence of the one professionally entitled to represent Mind. To speak is a razor-edged boomerang that lashes at your tongue without pause. The psychoanalytic police congregate like Rosenfeld's (1971) mobsters in the claustrophobic caverns of the psyche (Meltzer, 1990), where bodies know too much of the mind's rest. Kudos to Muriel for breaking the silence of the too muchness (Stein, 1998) as it is institutionalized in the conditions of our impossible profession. Her paper gives words to our collective muteness "regarding psychoanalysis' collective dilemma: the primal crime of sexual transgression" (Dimen, 2011a, p. 39).

Lapsus Linguae has been generative precisely because it opens the question of how boundary violation may be endemic to psychoanalytic work. Examining a symptom that heretofore registered as diagnostic of structural pathology in the analyst, analysand, or dyad, Muriel asks whether the symptom may in fact be structural to psychoanalysis itself. Our attention branches out from self-referential preoccupation with the terminology of the unconscious and liberal concern for the suffering Other to an ethical inquiry into the structure of analytic relationships in therapeutic dyads, in Institutes and guilds, among generations, and between these various bodies and the various ways that reified "frames" (Bass, 2007, 2008) and perverse boundary violations authorize minds without necessarily establishing a secure ground for ethical practice.

Late in his life, Winnicott (1988) described *the soul* as a space separate from the personality and from the punitive (and often self-punitive) fantasy that the mind resides in a singular place in the person such as the head or an integrative quality such as the intellect. Rather, soulful minds gather in a "specialized part of the psyche that is not necessarily body-linked" (p. 53). Maturity, he wrote, "means, among other things, a capacity for tolerating ideas, and parents need this capacity" (p. 59) to distinguish "between the child's dream (about erotic boundaries) and fact." This boundary establishes our mutual co-construction of belief (Aron, 1996) and sexuality (Corbett, 2009; Dimen, 1999). It must be violated so that fantasy may garner *respect,* a kind of knowledge with consequence that manifests in an effort to probe the boundary between separate subjects whose souls merit our collective concern. "Fantasy," Winnicott then commented, "in this way proves to be the human characteristic, the stuff of socialization and of civilization itself" (p. 60). Butler (1993, p. 267) aptly added that, "fantasy in this sense is to be understood not as an activity *of* an already informed subject, but the staging and dispersion of the subject into a variety of identificatory positions" in an array of desiring.

I am arguing that desire is a soulful and soul-wrenching, polymorphous quality of the spontaneous gesture in an emergent "self," when this self comes in contact with *the rest*. The sexual "self" is a transitional, potential phenomenon that is, by necessity homeless lest it be taken to possess a quality of "truth" that too often "murders" the soul. As Salamon writes (2010, p. 33), the vague material of sexuality "is always a precipitate of a psychic relation between body and world." When the emergent subject is proscribed, repressed, suppressed, or ridiculed, and the soul becomes the subject of Truth rather than the subject of fantasy (Levin, 2015), boundaries demarcate the Law in advance of transitional representation in embodied gestures.

The fate of this necessary crossing only becomes a disciplinary structure when the phantasmatic scene interpellates the subject as worthy of the object's censure. Hence my puzzling title, *when the body knows the mind's rest*, can be interpreted in a variety of ways that tender both certainty and doubt about several essentially contested pairings that occupy this Cartesian binary: is there a body without a mind? To whom(s) does it belong? Does the mind ever rest among other bodies? And if not, just how Other are they? Can there be relation without encounter or reverie without difference? I suggest that the problem we must address is not boundary violations per se but, rather, perverse boundary mis-violations that structure mute object relations among subjects in "the field" as disciplinary pairings; the muteness that characterizes these perverse boundary violations has a quality of obviousness (Althusser, 1971) that must be "resisted" in the analytic dyad for psychoanalysis to matter (Guralnik and Simeon, 2010).

I want to use *Lapsus Linguae* to describe the violation as representative of a structural condition in the matrix of inter-embodied communication that becomes perverse in *effect* when discourse about boundary violations is muted (psychically or institutionally) in service of discipline (Foucault, 1979). If this statement seems to dismiss the subject's need for an autonomous, impermeable boundary or Self in positing a kind of necessary violation, consider that unrequited desire (see *amae*, in Doi, 1989; Hartman, 2012; Taniguchi, 2012) has been understood to be a necessary violation of the erotic aim that penetrates the psyche-soma in a way that enables the subject's mindfulness of the collective *rest*. The ego requires the object in order to represent the superego, and since there can be no object relation without a social relation, there can be no field and no boundary without *the rest*. Unrequited desire, Muriel writes in one of the most breathtaking passages in *Lapsus Linguae*, "permits you to sense your desire as distinct from, other to, the desire of the other who matters to you as much as your own life. But you need someone else to help you do it (p. 61)."

In this eloquent twist of Jessica Benjamin's (1988; 1995) Hegelian maxim that, in the moment when one is recognized by the other, one is dependent on the other for recognition, Dimen exhibits longing: "Desire is about longing, not having. It may be sweet or poignant or terrible. But without it, one is as without appetite" (p. 51). We rely on the other to hold our desire in mind as representation—but not as fact. Desire collects in the symbolization of this violation, not in its realization (Lacan, 1977). The mind does flip flops when words are not yet ready to describe what the body already knows of the mind's longing for sensual recognition that crosses the boundary of the Other's *psyche-soma*. Tongues get confused when this violation is reified by action (Ferenczi, 1949); eyes cast a downward pall over an inward sense of abjection or worse, tongues wag in Institutional settings so that the *system* (representative of the *Discipline*) may punish the perpetrator as not-me but *one-of-the-rest* without taking a good look at its *own* constructed Self (Burka, 2008).

Tongues in motion

Indeed, psychoanalysis pays significant attention to how bodies are arranged in spatial relations to one another. As a requirement for membership in the guild, bodies must meet couch to chair. When bodies meet face-to-face, the interaction is deemed lesser. The increasing use of videoconferencing online has been met with the charge that bodies that are not in the same room can only parody relatedness because there is no *frame* (an abstraction that resides in the role of the analyst (Bleger, 1967) and therefore no pairing of container with contained (Cartwright, 2010). The analyst's body in an office convenes the field or the *beta screen* that allows masturbation fantasies to have generative potential that the computer screen is seen to lack (Caparrotta and Lemma, 2014; Galatzer-Levy, 2012). Erotic transference spatialized in a way that is sanctioned by the discipline is deemed generative. When it is spatialized in other ways, it is deemed perverse or pornographic. How is it that we have rendered the space of bodies alongside one another so necessary to the way we think about the mind yet for all our attention to the dance of attunement, we have so little theory of the choreography of bodies in the intersubjective choreography of mind (Chassay, 2015; Lepecki, 2013)? Perhaps this lacuna in psychoanalytic theorizing stems from the subtle challenge that attends any choreography: the audience.

The audience to the interaction of bodies and minds is always already defined by a plurality of Others, that is, by *the rest*. This mob of scrutinizing Others (mother and father in the primal scene; the internal panopticon represented as the "superego") was transformed by Kleinian thinkers into a phantasmatic grouping of split-off qualities of the self that responds to a primary terror (Rosenfeld, 1971; Steiner, 1993). The audience to boundary violations occupies a space of infinite internal regress such that the speaker can only describe violation as an impingement by the self on the self. Bion (1962) warned analytic candidates not to see it any other way if they care to decode the psyche. Only in recent work on transgenerational transmission of trauma within psychoanalysis (Harris and Kuchuck, 2015), normative unconscious processes (Layton, 2006), and the role of interpellation in the construction of the subject (Guralnik and Simeon, 2010) is power conceptualized beyond the purely internal scene of a fantasy or a particular relationship to cast bodies in motion.

We end up isolated from others who need to also test the boundaries that proffer desire but who may, by virtue of fear or contempt or lust or position or some rage of their own, disavow the violation inherent in desire and treat it not as an inter-embodied, symbolic communication of "the dream" of erotic awakening (Winnicott, 1988, p. 59), but as if it were a concrete request. I would call this a perverse boundary mis-violation. In life, as in psychoanalytic theories that fail to acknowledge the collective nature of erotic striving, it perpetuates an odd splitting of the body from mind's rest. Boundaries that are spatialized in rhythmic exchange between bodies other than those legislated by compulsory heterosexuality or deemed appropriate aspects of maternality (Sheehy, 2012) become appended to the subject's relationship with the object as a mental investment in a particular object relation when they might rather be understood as moments in the elaboration of the psyche-soma. Boundaries, said another way, become characteristic of internal object relations at the expense of the articulate choreography of bodies in the expansive field of sexuality.

When the boundary aspect appended to the introject is *unspeakable*, it lurks as a deficit in the analysand awaiting repair. Since the boundary appended to the transference object lurks in the patient at the privilege of the analyst, it is the analyst's responsibility to extricate the analytic subject from this burden by first making reparation for his or her countertransference wish for the boundary to be breached by the patient. As I recently wrote paying homage to no less a boundary violator than Masud Khan (Hartman, 2013b, p. 416; Khan, 1989), "by holding the double meaning of countertransference, as discourse between patient and analyst that allows for affect to be contained and represented and as a way of knowing endowed by the analyst's occupation of normative discourse, the analyst has the opportunity to coax the patient into the domain of representation." When the burden of *the rest* thus migrates from the patient to the analyst and back again, the violation can be shared and approached as a matter of thick description (Geertz, 1973) rather than pathology.

This is the meaning of Dimen's (2001) exquisite title: *Perversion is Us.* Only when *prolonged echoes mingling in the distance* (Baudelaire, 1954) emanate from the forest of pre-presented symbols can a perverse mis-violation of the boundary be represented in the analytic dyad. Otherwise, it rests mute and it mutates. An analyst such as Dr. O bestows upon us the illegitimacy of our desire in a manner that conforms with the *obvious* priority of the analytic field to demand the patient speak. His silence (and the atmosphere of complicity guaranteed by his professional stature) links an enduring attack on the patient's need to represent the soul to the body to our poker-faced shame because, in Dr O's economy, it is the patient who must speak.

Arguing against this perverse logic, Khan wrote (1989, p. 17), "the ana-lyst has to make the reparation so that differentiated personalization can begin to operate." Whether it is voiced or articulated without voice among the negotiators of a liminal zone (McGleughlin, 2015b), repar-ation of this sort allows itinerant desire a home in the body. This is the heroic task that Dimen (2011a) set for herself. So, if I may replace Dimen's word "parent" with the enjoined "analyst," we find in Dimen's text a credo with which to chart passage through the thicket of boundary violations necessary and perverse:

> You need to be able to experience your desire, abject and soar-ing, with your analyst who is feeling this too and knows it and is intentionally not acting but is instead bearing the poignant sight of your passion as it bursts into flame, you with whom your analyst has identified, who she or he identifies as her or his own, and who she or he is allowing to live"
>
> (p. 61)

Me and Angel down by the schoolyard

Years ago, back when the field that our bodies groped in was framed by the ever-present specter of viral contamination, my patient's tongue landed in my lap. I shared the experience in a group supervision at work and was accused of a sexual boundary violation. Nothing came of it, thank God, other than a lot of sleep-less nights and dreams of exile to analytic hell.

I had a patient who was dying. I'll call him Angel. He must have been an incredible hunk, Angel, before his body began to wither. I was working on an AIDS ward doing consultation-liaison. Physicians, say what you will, are not able to deal with bodies. They float through medical rounds in military phalanx dissociated from the embodied experience of their patients. My job, as I understood it, was to translate the felt sense of the patient's body to the obdurate diagnostician.

I'll keep it short, because the amount of ooze is gross when, day after day, you move among them dying of Plague. Angel and I connected in some way that I can't quite explain. He was a straight drug addict from the Bronx and me an eager to contribute downtown gay. We met five times a week for one year until his death.

One day, while Angel was particularly weak and his lungs hosted phlegm so full of bacteria that you could practically watch the writhing of microbes through the screen of his skin, I was at his bedside on the ICU. I had just returned from London where I'd observed how Anna Freud's couch positioned her patients' heads just inches from her lap. The configuration of hospital gurney and nursing stool was similarly familiar. Angel was telling me a story, I don't recall about what, and a slice of his desiccated tongue flew out of his mouth and landed in my lap. I popped a hard-on.

It's an extreme story. I don't mean to be sensational. But it's true. I was ashamed and confused. Angel didn't seem to notice, but a pause in his breathing let me know that we shared an experience of erotic terror. Angel was ruined for sex. He would never sire children. And me? I felt so confused and guilty about my erection that I sprinted to supervision. Thanks to my consultants, Maria Derevenko and John Budin, I was able to think about the confluence of erotics, body integrity, the death instinct, survival, narcissism, and just plain love. And to feel it too.

Angel died soon after. We never touched in a sexual way, although I held his hand a few times when he was delirious. When they took Angel's body from the room, after his family left, I sat in the room for an hour alone. Have you ever had a Reiki massage? It felt like that.

The charge of sexual boundary violation came later, in a different hospital, on a psychiatric dual diagnosis ward populated with AIDS patients, from a nurse who was pretending not to be homophobic while dispensing "the AIDS cocktail" to addicts as if it were a reward for good behavior—like methadone in a rehab. We had sparred over her disciplinary tactics. I was not kind when, during a series of layoffs, Nurse Ratchet's seniority in the union forced her promotion and the sacking of our beloved nurse, a lesbian single mother who had earlier been *outed* and dishonorably discharged from the US Army.

Nurse Ratchet was out to get me, and when I told the story of me and Angel and the flight of the tongue, she found a way. "I was trying to silence her" by bringing to our supervision group a *sickening* tale of sexual excess. Was I? Indeed, in my most frightened moments on my analyst's couch dreaming up a legal nightmare, I wondered if she were right. I had told the story of Angel with a certain arrogance. Perhaps showing off? I recall wanting to help my younger colleagues feel empowered to swim in the beta swamp of AIDS panic with their psychotic patients. Empowering as in "allowing," as in "allowing to live" or "allowing to think" or "allowing to feel" is where we analysts get tripped up. Fantasy is not always empowering.

Dr O. seems to have imagined that he was *empowering* Dimen to live. Ultimately, she felt his patrician bestowal of permission as intensely as his hard-on. *Empowering* inevitably brings us to the level of the allow-er and the allow-ee: a doer and done to snare if ever there was one (Benjamin, 2004). In this regard, Dimen is very wise to note that boundary violations are best addressed as a collective responsibility. The boundaries each of us must violate circulate among the rest. Contra Bleger's (1967) location of the frame in the empowering role of the analyst, the frame resides among us and alongside the rest. We frame; we must therefore address perverse boundary violations as a collective matter. Codes of individual ethical conduct do not apply to disciplinary amassing of power (even if the US Supreme Court would have us treat corporations as if individual citizens). Nor do proceedings against errant souls collectively acquit members of the guild. Insofar as we squelch a social, ethical instinct to query context and we revert to the psychoanalytic default position of analyzing the damaged individual, we mute the field.

Nurse Ratchet and I fell into a perverse boundary violation because the reality of homophobic employment practices could not be named in a unionized field. At the same time, perhaps I was allowing myself to intrude in the Other mind's rest? Had I committed the crime of Dr O? Did I imagine that I knew better and could protect and empower more? Had I fed Nurse Ratchet the lexicon of my own unresolved boundary violation with Angel and used it to silence her? As Dimen explains quite succinctly: "Analysts suffering the dissociated, *unforgettable abjection of having been patients* may indeed find themselves inducing that very feeling in their own patients (colleagues), in order to cleanse themselves and, thus cleansed, to become pure and strong" (Dimen, 2011a, p. 73, emphasis and parens added).

I was stronger than Angel. I had a boner. He had a shredded tongue. I was weaker than Nurse Ratchet. I had a boner. She had a union contract. I was stronger than Nurse Ratchet: I am a psychoanalyst. We could go back and forth till doomsday assigning blame and winning a reprieve in the interest of recovering from the unforgettable abjection of having been *analysts* (Ghent, 1992). As, I suppose, we must.

Notes

1 Many thanks to Charles Levin, whose remarkable editorial guidance was with me through the writing of this paper plus all the rest that came with it.
2 Indeed, there is a way of reading Winnicott that reduces transitional phenomena to "uniquely field-dependent phenomena" (Peltz and Goldberg, 2013). However, from my perspective in reading Winnicott, contemporary theorizations of a generalized, uniquely analytic "field" would seem rather more like omnipotent fantasies (on the part of the analytic theoretician) who is impatient with transitionality and wishes to gain control over its uncertain fate in culture and the intersubjective relationship by diminishing its social valence.
3 See Bersani, 2010 and Bersani and Phillips, 2010, for a discussion of psychoanalytic "correspondences" between the shattering of the self and its accretion in solidarity with liminal subjects.
4 In an implicit critique of object relations, Schilder imagines a situation where a social condition among bodies might lead someone to evacuate a whole object, i.e. the "self." This seems to me an important insight into how "cruising" and other collective erotic geographies gel among desiring subjects.
5 See for example, Butler (1995) on melancholy gender-refused identification.
6 This is one of the great benefits of the use of avatars by discomfited souls online. The body's capacity for re-signification allows it to find a space in the online user's mind. This has been especially true for transgender people who find no ready home for the mind in traditionally gendered bodies.

References

Althusser, L. (1971). *Lenin and philosophy and other essays.* New York: Monthly Review Press.
Aron, L. (1996). *A meeting of minds.* Hillsdale, NJ: Analytic Press.
Asibong, A. (2015). "Then look!" Unborn attachments and the half-moving image. *Studies in Gender and Sexuality,* 16: 87–102.
Baranger, M. and Baranger, W. (2008). The analytic situation as a dynamic field. *International Journal of Psychoanalysis,* 89: 795–826.

Bass, A. (2007). When the frame doesn't fit the picture. *Psychoanalytic Dialogues*, 17: 1–27.

Bass, A. (2008). A Few more thoughts on the frame: Forms, functions, and meanings. *Psychoanalytic Dialogues*, 18: 262–268.

Baudelaire, C. (1954). *The flowers of evil*. W. Aggeler, trans. Fresno, CA: Academic Library Guild.

Benjamin, J. (1988). *The bonds of love*. New York: Pantheon.

Benjamin, J. (1995). *Like subjects, love objects*. New Haven, CT: Yale University Press.

Benjamin, J. (2004). Beyond doer and done to: An intersubjective view of thirdness. *Psychoanalytic Quarterly*, 73: 5–46.

Bersani, L. (2010). *Is the rectum a grave? and other Essays*. Chicago, IL: University of Chicago Press.

Bersani, L. and Phillips, A. (2010). *Intimacies*. Chicago, IL: University of Chicago Press.

Bhabha, H. (1994). *The location of culture*. New York: Routledge.

Bion, W.R. (1962). *Learning from experience*. London, UK: Heinmann.

Bleger, J. (1967). Psycho-analysis of the psycho-analytic frame. *International Journal of Psychoanalysis*, 48: 511–519.

Burka, J.B. (2008). Psychic fallout from breach of confidentiality. *Contemporary Psychoanalysis*, 44: 177–198.

Butler, J. (1993). *Bodies that matter: On the discursive limits of "sex"*. New York: Routledge.

Butler, J. (1995). Melancholy gender: Refused identification. *Psychoanalytic Dialogues*, 5: 165–180.

Caparrotta, L. and Lemma, A. (2014). Introduction. In: L. Caparrotta and A. Lemma (Eds.), *Psychoanalysis in the technoculture era*. New York: Routledge, pp. 1–22.

Carnochan, P. (2001). *Looking for ground: Countertransference and the problem of value in psychoanalysis*. New York: Routledge.

Cartwright, D. (2010). *Containing states of mind*. New York: Routledge.

Chassay, S. (2015). Tis beauty killed the beast. *Studies in Gender and Sexuality*, 16: 5–17.

Corbett, K. (2009). *Boyhoods*. New Haven, CT: Yale University Press.

Deleuze, G. and Guattari, F. (1977). *Anti-Oedipus: Capitalism and Schizophrenia*. Trans. R. Hurley, M. Seem, & H.R. Lane. New York: Viking.

Deleuze, G. and Guattari, F. (1987). *A Thousand Plateaus: Capaitalism and Schizophrenia*. Trans. Brian Massumi. Minneapolis: University of Minnesota Press.

Dimen, M. (1991). Deconstructing difference: Gender, splitting, and transitional space. *Psychoanalytic Dialogues*, 1: 335–352.

Dimen, M. (1999). Between lust and libido: Sex, psychoanalysis, and the moment before. *Psychoanalytic Dialogues*, 9: 415–440.

Dimen, M. (2000). The body as rorschach. *Studies in Gender and Sexuality*, 1: 9–39.

Dimen, M. (2001). Perversion is us? *Psychoanalytic Dialogues*, 11: 825–860.

Dimen, M. (2005). Sexuality and suffering, Or the eew! factor. *Studies in Gender and Sexuality*, 6: 1–18.

Dimen, M. (2011a). Lapsus linguae, or a slip of the tongue? *Contemporary Psychoanalysis*, 47: 35–79.

Dimen, M. (2011b). With culture in mind: The social third. Introduction: Writing the clinical and the social. *Studies in Gender and Sexuality*, 12: 1–3.

Dimen, M. (2014). Inside the revolution: Power, sex, and technique in Freud's "'Wild' Analysis". *Psychoanalytic Dialogues*, 24: 499–515.

Dimen, M. and Goldner, V. (2002). *Gender in psychoanalytic space*. New York: Other Press.

Doi, T. (1989). The concept of amae and its psychoanalytic implications. *International Review of Psycho-Analysis*, 16: 349–354.

Dor, J. (1999). *The clinical Lacan*. New York: Other Press.

Ferenczi, S. (1949). Confusion of tongues between the adults and the child— (The language of tenderness and passion. *International Journal of Psycho-analysis*, 30: 225–230.

Ferro, A. (2009). *The analytic field: A clinical concept*. London, UK: Karnac Books.

Foucault, M. (1977). *The history of sexuality, Volume 1: An introduction*. New York: Pantheon Books.

Foucault, M. (1979). *Discipline and punish*. New York: Vintage Books.

Foucault, M. (1980). *Power/Knowledge*. New York: Pantheon Books.

Foucault, M. (1986). Of other spaces. *Diacritics*, 16(1): 22–27.

Freud, S. (1923/1961). The ego and the id. In: J. Strachey (Ed. & Trans.), *The complete psychological works of Sigmund Freud* (Vol. 19). London: Hogarth, pp. 3–66.

Galatzer-Levy, R.M. (2012). Obscuring desire: A special pattern of male adolescent masturbation. *Psychoanalytic Inquiry*, 32: 480–495.

Geertz, C. (1973). *The interpretation of cultures*. New York: Basic Books.

Gerson, S. (2011). Hysteria and humiliation. *Psychoanalytic Dialogues*, 21: 517–530.

Ghent, E. (1990). Masochism, submission, surrender: Masochism as a perversion of surrender. *Contemporary Psychoanalysis*, 26: 108–136.

Ghent, E. (1992). Paradox and process. *Psychoanalytic Dialogues*, 2: 135–159.

Goldberg, P. (2012). Active perception and the search for sensory symbiosis. *JAPA*, 60: 791–812.

Gonzalez, F.J. (2012). Loosening the bonds: Psychoanalysis, feminism, and the problem of the group. *Studies in Gender and Sexuality*, 13(4): 253–267.

Green, A. (1975). The Analyst, symbolization and absence in the analytic setting (On changes in analytic practice and analytic experience)—In memory of D. W. Winnicott. *International Journal of Psychoanalysis*, 56: 1–22.

Guralnik, O. (2011). Ede: Race, the Law, and I. *Studies in Gender and Sexuality*, 12: 22–26.

Guralnik, O. and Simeon, D. (2010). Depersonalization: Standing in the spaces between recognition and interpellation. *Psychoanalytic Dialogues*, 20: 400–416.

Harris, A. and Kuchuck, S. (2015). *The legacy of Sandor Ferenczi: From ghost to ancestor*. New York: Routledge.

Hartman, S. (2010). *L'état c'est moi*, except when I am not: Commentary on paper by Orna Gurlnik and Daphne Simeon. *Psychoanalytic Dialogues*, 20: 428–436.

Hartman, S. (2012). Of mothers and other collective lovers: Inspired by Kyoko Taniguchi's "The eroticism of the maternal: So what if everything is about the mother?". *Studies in Gender and Sexuality*, 13(2): 139–144.

Hartman, S. (2013a). On viability and indebtedness—Or, "get away from her you bitch!" Commentary on Simon's "Spoken through desire". *Studies in Gender and Sexuality*, 14: 309–317.

Hartman, S. (2013b). On making reparation to the analyst's idolized countertransference. Commentary on paper by Dana Amir. *Psychoanalytic Dialogues*, 23: 408–417.

Hoffman, I. (1983). The patient as interpreter of the analyst's experience. *Contemporary Psychoanalysis*, 19: 389–422.

Khan, M.M. (1989). *Alienation in perversions*. London, UK: Karnac Books.

Kristeva, J. (1995). *New maladies of the soul*. New York: Columbia University Press.

Lacan, J. (1977). *Ecrits. (Trans. A. Sheridan)*. New York: Norton.

Laplanche, J. (1999). *Essays on Otherness*. New York: Routledge.

Laplanche, J. (2003/2011). Gender, sex, and the sexual. In: J. Fletcher (Ed.), *Freud and the sexual: Essays 2000–2006*. New York: International Psychoanalytic Books, pp. 159–202.

Layton, L. (2006). Attacks on linking: The unconscious pull to dissociate individuals from their social context. In L. Layton, S. Gatwell and N. Hollander (Eds.), *Class and politics: Encounters in the clinical setting*. London, UK: Routledge, pp. 107–117.

Lepecki, A. (2013). Teleplastic abduction: Subjectivity in the age of ART, or delirium and psychoanalysis: Commentary on Simon's "Spoken Through Desire.". *Studies in Gender and Sexuality*, 14: 300–309.

Levin, C. (2015). Personal communication.

McGleughlin, J. (2015a). Do we find or lose ourselves in the negative? *Psychoanalytic Dialogues*, 25(2): 214–236.

McGleughlin, J. (2015b). Answering gestures. *Psychoanalytic Dialogues*, 25(2): 256–264.

Meltzer, D. (1990). *The claustrum: An investigation of claustrophobic phenomena*. London: Karnac Books.

Ogden, T.H. (2004). On holding and containing, being and dreaming. *International Journal of Psychoanalysis*, 85: 1349–1364.

Peltz, R. and Goldberg, P. (2013). Field conditions: Discussion of Donnel B. Stern's "Field theory in psychoanalysis". *Psychoanalytic Dialogues*, 23: 660–666.

Rosenfeld, H. (1971). A Clinical approach to the psychoanalytic theory of the life and death instincts: An Investigation into the aggressive aspects of narcissism. *International Journal of Psychoanalysis*, 52: 169–178.

Rundel, M. (2015). The Fire of Eros: Sexuality and the Movement Toward Union. *Psychoanalytic Dialogues*, 25(5): 614–630.

Sakeketopoulou, A. (2014). To suffer pleasure: The shattering of the ego as the psychic labor of perverse sexuality. *Studies in Gender and Sexuality*, 15: 254–268.

Salamon, G. (2010). *Assuming a body: Transgender and rhetorics of materiality*. New York: Columbia University Press.

Scarfone, D. (2015). *The unpast: The actual unconscious*. Trans. D. Bonnigal-Katz. New York: UIT Books.

Schilder, P. (1950). *The image and appearance of the human body*. New York: International Universities Press.

Sheehy, M. (2012). Sparring with the eternal maternal abject. *Studies in Gender and Sexuality*, 13: 65–87.

Stein, R. (1998). The enigmatic dimension of sexual experience: The "otherness" of sexuality and primal seduction. *Psychoanalytic Quarterly*, 67(594): 625.

Stein, R. (2005). Why perversion? False love and the perverse pact. *International Journal of Psychoanalysis*, 86: 775–799.

Stein, R. (2007). Laplanche's theory of sexuality. *Studies in Gender and Sexuality*, 8: 177–2000.

Steiner, J. (1993). *Psychic retreats: Pathological organisations of the personality in psychotic, neurotic, and borderline patients*. London and New York: Routledge.

Stern, D.B. (2013). Field theory in psychoanalysis, part 2: Bionian field theory and contemporary interpersonal/relational psychoanalysis. *Psychoanalytic Dialogues*, 23: 630–645.

Taniguchi, K. (2012). The eroticism of the maternal: So what if everything is about the mother? *Studies in Gender and Sexuality*, 13(2): 123–138.

Turner, V. (1967). Betwixt and between: The liminal period in rites of passage. In *The Forest of Symbols*. Ithaca, NY: Cornell University Press.

Winnicott, D.W. (1951). Transitional objects and transitional phenomena—A Study of the first not-me possession. *International Journal of Psychoanalysis*, 34: 89–97.

Winnicott, D.W. (1958). The capacity to be alone. *International Journal of Psychoanalysis*, 39: 416–420.

Winnicott, D.W. (1971). *Playing and Reality*. London, UK: Tavistock.

Winnicott, D.W. (1988). *Human Nature*. New York: Patheon Books.

Chapter 9

From no to know
Charting the "Space Between"

Ann Pellegrini

In his introduction to *Wild Analysis*, a new translation of Freud's collected papers on technique, Adam Phillips describes psychoanalysis as "about what two people can say to each other if they agree not to have sex" (2002, p. xx). I love this description of psychoanalysis, and love may be all to the point. Elsewhere, Phillips posits the "analytic relation as [proffering] a vital clue to new forms of loving outside the analytic situation" (2008, p. 92). In this picture of things, psychoanalysis is at once a way of practicing love, in the sense of practicing for it elsewhere (a different kind of "other scene"), and *already* love practiced and desire learned.

And yet, as Muriel Dimen so poignantly narrates in *Lapsus linguae* (2011a), renunciation is no simple matter. Not only does eroticism pulse through the analytic exchange, via transferences and counter-transferences, but all too often sexual boundaries between chair and couch are literally breached. Sexual transgressions are an open secret, "the primal crime that we have not solved," as Dimen writes (p. 73). That everyone knows this has generally not produced curiosity, how-ever—let alone soul-searching. Instead there come the inward turn of shame and a tongue-tied self-censorship: "We do not ... want this crime and our knowledge of it to be public, either among ourselves or the laity, lest we risk the shame that shames" (p. 73).

Everyone knows and yet no one speaks. So Dimen risks her own shaming shame in telling her personal story of a sexual violation that occurred in the course of a long treatment with Dr. O, the *nom de divan* she assigns her analyst. She reports that in one particularly exasperating session, she literally overturned Dr. O's couch.

If a couch falls in the consulting room, does it make any sound?

The reddened face of shame that Dimen presents to her readers, and for a broader psychoanalytic community, gives a different hue to Phillips' rosy picture of the analytic scene. Nonetheless, as Dimen herself concludes, "psychoanalysis deserves to be construed beyond idealization and demonization" (p. 75). And between these two poles lies the messy territory of an encounter between two positions—analyst and patient—neither of which unfolds from a place of purity.

One of the many important interventions made by Dimen in her essay is to remind other analysts that they have all been patients themselves, at least once. Because of this, they necessarily bring their own experience as patients into the clinical encounter. The analyst's mixed position—"these two self-states," Dimen calls them (p. 71)—no doubt contributes, however unconsciously, to the power dynamics enacted in treatment.

Power differentials structure the analytic relationship; they are not peculiar to the O/Dimen dyad. Too often, however, analysts forget what it felt like to be a patient and to play bottom to the analyst's top. Of course, there is forgetting and there is forgetting. Dimen speculates that the shame of laying oneself bare on a couch before the ears and eyes of another shadows an analyst's counter-transferences. In particular, she wonders if the "dissociated, unforgettable abjection" of being a patient is sometimes (regularly?) transferred—dumped, really—by an analyst onto his or her patient (p. 73). When gender's additional contributions to the layering of power between analyst and analysand are active, but un- or under-analyzed, the possibility of going off the rails increases exponentially. Dumping may take an explicitly sexual form, with the analyst seeking to recuperate the power given up when he (or she) was once a patient. As Dimen herself puts it in a tentative phrasing that wavers between question and answer, "Maybe this explosive combination of power and shame in the analyst/patient hierarchy has something to do with why sexual betrayal of patients by analysts is a systemic hazard: it has nowhere to go but up and out" (pp. 72–3).

Or does it?

If Dimen calls attention to the "two self-states alive" in the analyst, with their mixture of power and abjection, she does so because she believes critical reflection on and *from* the place of this doubleness might be a resource for developing a different kind of "space between" (p. 71). Negotiating and inhabiting this space will require thinking about gender and thinking about sex, albeit on altered terms. For Dimen, this means that we need to place sex in a relational context. Her re-contextualization of the place and meaning of "the sexual" in an individual's development problematizes our understanding of the Oedipal drama. The relationship between analytic theory and ethics is undermined and transformed by Dimen's reconsideration of the tasks and responsibilities of the analyst who is cast *in loco parentis*.

Dimen's fascinating "three-dimensional relational theory" (p. 74) of the incest prohibition introduces a crucial separation between Oedipus and the incest taboo. By the former, she means those tasks of individuation necessary to the child, who must distinguish her own desires from her parents and do so in this double sense. The child must renounce desire for the parent/s (just say no), and she must separate her desire from theirs so as to lay claim to her own desires and *ways* of desiring. This latter task—*just say know?* (and let's preserve that question mark, which is all to the point)—is about more than saying yes to sex. After all, the Oedipus complex imagines that there is a right kind of no and a right kind of yes to say when it comes to sex. Desire is far bigger and messier than Oedipus. So is psychoanalysis. How to develop a language of affirming sexual desire and sexual pleasure beyond or, if this is impossible, beside Oedipus and "with culture in mind," to use the title of Dimen's recent volume (2011b)? Not only that, but how to develop critical vocabularies and critical practices that do not mystify the power relations that Oedipal assumptions bring into the room?

As Orna Guralnik observes in the online IARPP Forum dedicated to Dimen's essay, "the profession structures its prohibitions to resonate with the incest taboo, and thus invites the participants to revisit an Oedipal scene … as a kind of hypnotic induction" (2011). Put otherwise: the structuring bar of Oedipus organizes the analytic relation as prohibition and lure at once. Saying "no" to the patient generates and may even mandate some kinds of self-knowing while blocking some others. Psychoanalysis is thus a practice of disciplinary power, in the sense meant by Foucault (1978, 1979). Disciplinary power refers to the array of institutional and cultural practices that have produced individuals *as* individuals, investing them—investing us—with particular beliefs about and commitment to their inner selves, the core of their beings. Disciplinary power does not do its work on pre-existing individuals; it is rather the method through which the experience of being a particular kind of individual takes shape. The disciplines are not primarily methods of correction or punishment, though they are also that. They are fundamentally productive: methods of power that organize behavior, normalize individuals, and generate a sense of bounded interiority. In western modernity, this interiority has been crucially embedded—"produced"—by discourses of sexuality and the disciplinary practices that teach us that sex is at our core, an argument extensively presented in the first volume of Foucault's *History of Sexuality* (1978). The original French title of this text better summarizes his argument concerning the way discourses of "sex" and "sexuality" conduct power: *La Volonté de savoir* (1976), usually translated as "the will to knowledge."

Foucault presents psychoanalysis as the paradigmatic secular site for the disciplinary production of modern sexuality: we confess our sins no longer to God's intermediary; we now spill out our secrets to ears for pay. But there is always more. If our secrets are un-ending, because unknown even or, even primarily, to ourselves, then the need for speech and self-knowledge is endless too. Enter Oedipus. No exit. The Oedipal scene is simultaneously incubator of the sexuality that is to come, warden over it, and lurking threat. This is so in the family cell projected through Oedipal desires and anxieties; it is also the case in the analytic room, insofar as not openly resembling Oedipus (or Jocasta) is the guiding rule from no to know. If, in some (most?) versions of psychoanalysis the Oedipal frame always structures the room, perhaps the best to be hoped for is not to seem too much like Oedipus (or Jocasta): not not-Oedipus, not not-Jocasta. These are tricky knots indeed.

But, what other reasons for not crossing the erotic boundary line with a patient could be ventured, which would *not* reproduce the Oedipal family as starting place and endpoint for sexual identity and sexual difference—or psychoanalysis, for that matter? Psychoanalysis is also or could also be a place where we (analysts and patients) get to practice creative un-knowing together, including creatively un-knowing what "sex" is or does or could be. But the profession's preferred analogies may block some of this creativity. When analysts call "on each other to behave like (good) parents" and "abstain from sexual action" with a patient (Dimen, 2011a, p. 75), good parenting or bad, there is little chance of Oedipus leaving the room. Could other critical concepts crack the door open? I am not arguing that we can avoid talking about parents or parenting. But I am pushing against doing it through the prism of Oedipus.

I hear Dimen taking an important step in this direction via the distinction she draws between Oedipus and the incest taboo. Although this is not Dimen's explicit interest in her article, the distinction has major implications for the queer or proto-gay child. For such a child, the project of differentiating her or his desires from the mimeticism expected of her by parents and a wider culture may be especially difficult and, even, traumatic. This is so because the expectation cum demand that "my" child grow up to be heterosexual just like the "me" or the "us" of the parents arguably recuperates incestuous parental desires *for* the child by issuing a demand *to* the child for sexual fidelity: to wit, grow up to desire as I do, heterosexually. The increasing social and legal acceptance of homosexuality and same-sex marriage may generate its own straight-jacketing normativities: grow up to desire as *we* do, *maritally.*

A parent's incestuous desires can thus be materialized in multiple forms, through corporeal violation, yes, but also through the delimitation of a child's imaginative horizons: a narrowing of the possible I's that child might take on and keep becoming over a lifetime. This is why Dimen's move to address the incest taboo to adults is so crucial. Adults are better positioned than the child to renounce the realization of their desires and hold the other's needs in mind without experiencing these twin tasks as erasing the self (p. 57). On the contrary, the "adults in charge" might even experience this "juggling act," which does entail loss, as paradoxically "self-enhancing" (p. 57). The adults in charge are the parents, but this is a role and responsibility the analyst also takes on *among other roles and responsibilities.* Moreover, in an analytic context, the desires that must be renounced can themselves become an object of critical and shared self-reflection between analyst and patient.

In offering her provocative conceptual separation between Oedipus and the incest taboo (processes she yet recognizes as "concurrent and interpenetrating" [p. 57]), Dimen importantly nuances the aphorism from Adam Phillips with which I began: "psychoanalysis is about what two people can say to each other if they agree not to have sex." This is a great line and a wonderful fantasy, too, but Dimen shows us that it is not the *patient's* task or responsibility to agree not to have sex. In therapy, the analyst must be the "adult in charge" who says no and, in so doing, gently encourages the process of coming to know differently—a difference that includes the invitation not to know once and for all. To put a queer spin on Winnicott (1965), desire, including sexual desire, is not something lying around waiting to be found. It must be created, but on the patient's terms not the analyst's, and, I'd insist, without the presumption that there is a particular object (or identification) waiting to be found. Further, as Dimen reminds, the "no" of analytic renunciation is not all or only loss. It is the condition for new enunciations. This "two-person materialization of the incest prohibition" (p. 59) opens a space for the child or the patient to find her own way of desire, a path as prone to error and loss as to fulfillment. But they will be her own errors and losses, which is its own bittersweet achievement for child/patient and for parent/analyst, too.

I come to this essay not as an analyst, but as a professor of queer theory. (I'm also a patient who was once a child.) I mention my different institutional context not out of anxiety or, at least, not out of too much anxiety, but out of desire and curiosity to move across the disciplinary locations and discursive practices that too often and too easily separate clinicians from cultural theorists. Put differently, what might clinicians and cultural theorists say to and learn from each other if we agree not to have sects?

Certainly, there are numerous overlaps between the consulting room and the classroom. The following list is hardly exhaustive, but just for starters: in both spaces, imbalances in power are structured into the scene of exchange. However friendly and approachable a professor may appear, for example, ultimately she passes judgment on her students by grading them.[1] For their part, analysts may not give their patients actual grades (however much many patients may yearn for such a concrete marker of progress and change), but they do assess their patients, as when they assign diagnoses for the purposes of insurance and intake forms. Analysts also judge their patients (however much they may try not to). They may do so silently, aloud with a supervisor, or aloud to their patients. (Isn't this last a boundary violation, too?)

In both spaces, the "adult in charge" once sat in the other chair: all professors have been students, all analysts have been patients. Dimen stresses the importance, for analysts, of being alive to their own history as patients, so they may better witness patients' experiences of vulnerability and abjection. Professors, too, carry these two self-states within, and would thus do well to recall the insecurities, defensiveness, boredom, vulnerabilities, as well as the vertiginous pleasures of being a student. In contrast to Dimen's concern that analysts may too easily forget they were once patients, it seems to me that the professor's "counter-transference" may regularly take another form: we are liable to misrecognize our students as our own younger selves and attribute to them the same investments we once had (Pellegrini, 1999, p. 624). This misrecognition might result in acts of reparative tenderness or tough love.[2] But in either case, this kind of misrecognition can block recognizing what our students want or could want, if we gave them the space to want differently.

The incitement to speech is also the incitement to desire—and to knowledge. Both the classroom and the consulting room put their participants at the cliff's edge of new knowledges and experiences. What would it feel like to fall off? Are there any nets? One net is the analyst's rule against any sexual action. This seems like a good guideline for the classroom, too. But, supplementing Dimen, I would say that this abstinence is not simply about allowing patients (or children or students) to discover their own *sexual* desires and what these might mean for themselves, past, present, future. It is also, critically, about creating space to learn what else desire could mean other than a desire for sex. The swirl of desires, spoken and unspoken, in the consulting room and the classroom exceeds the desire for sex. Among the potential violences enacted through consensual sex between analyst and patient, or between professor and student, is the reduction of *eros* to sex. We need a thicker theory of desire and pleasure. Neither psychoanalysis nor feminist and queer cultural theories can do this on their own.

This is not a call for sublimation or the channeling of sexual desires and pleasures into licit, non-sexual forms. Quite the contrary: the privilege set on sex as epistemological and moral center of the individual can make it hard to see, recognize, and value other kinds of embodied and embodying desires and pleasures. The scene of pedagogy—and the classroom and the consulting room are both such scenes—overflows with desires and identifications irreducible to sex. Earlier I referred to the kinds of misrecognitions to which professors may be especially liable: mistaking our students for our own younger selves, perhaps even seeing in them the sorts of students who grew up to become professors, just like us. Identifications are cross-cut by desire: the desire to be easily converts into the desire to have. But the movement between being and having cannot be stopped without stopping pedagogy. It becomes all the more crucial, then, not to make sex the action or motive wish towards which desire points. Professors may well be the kind of student who kept falling in love in the classroom; love and desire for particular styles of thought or for a particular genre or historical period or for one very special author (ah, Jane! ah, Freud! ah, Plato!) may be what converted us (I'll own my own conversion narrative) from student to professor. And perhaps this conversion even passed through desire for a professor. But, as I have written elsewhere (Pellegrini, 1999), the student crush may itself trace "a desire for and identification with the professor's desire" for subject X or methodology Y. Neither the language of sexuality nor the language of Oedipal transmission does justice to this pedagogic scene of desire and identification. Pedagogy takes place at the join of identification and desire; it is cut through by the erotic. That does not mean it is about sex.

Certainly, the cultural and psychic confusion of desire with sex can lead to sexual boundary violations between faculty and student. Calling it pedagogy is no alibi.[3] For the purposes of this volume, I am not interested in debating the wisdom or ethics of consensual faculty-student sexual relations, about which there is already a large and still-growing literature (see, for example, Gallop, 1997; Kipnis, 2015; Wolf and Dolan, 1997). Instead, I am trying to initiate a conversation beyond law and taboo and perhaps beyond sex "itself" (whatever sex is). The primacy accorded sex—it is desire's privileged expression and injury's worst form—makes such conversations both difficult and all the more urgent.

The university precincts I traverse were roiled by heated debates from the mid-1980s onward over sexual boundary violations in the classroom, aka sexual harassment, and the question, could a student ever meaningfully consent to "amorous relations" (the euphemism employed by many a university sexual harassment policy) with her/his teacher. More recently, college campuses have been the site of impassioned and important debates over sexual assault. In many ways, these debates are heirs to the "sex wars" that riveted and divided feminists throughout the 1980s, and which Dimen knows something about first-hand. She was a speaker at the (in)famous 1982 Barnard College "Scholar and the Feminist" conference, which was organized around the topic of women's sexuality. Anti-pornography feminists picketed the conference and accused the invited speakers of promoting violence against women. Their crime? The speakers refused to cede the matter of sexual agency and instead asserted the complexity of women's erotic lives. They also refused a unified view of "woman" or "women." (Pluralizing woman to women did not then and does not now eliminate questions of difference.) While participants in this conference acknowledged the sexual dangers women faced (and face) in a patriarchal world, they also wanted to think aloud about the multiple forms women's sexual pleasures might take. The title of the now-classic conference volume—*Pleasure and Danger: Exploring Female Sexuality* (Vance, 1984)—captures something of the complexity the conference speakers variously addressed as well as the ambivalences owned up to. Dimen's own contribution to that volume (Dimen, 1984) wittily bespeaks a related and irresolvable ambivalence: "Politically Correct? Politically Incorrect?"

Pleasure *and* danger. Conjunctions are hard. They can be bumpy, even bruising. But we all do well to bear in mind the ongoing charge and challenge not to come down on one side of the binary: pleasure or danger; correct or incorrect; yes or no. As feminist and queer legal scholar Katherine Franke puts it, sounding more like an analyst than a lawyer,

> Desire is not subject to cleaning up, to being purged of its nasty, messy, perilous dimensions, full of contradictions and the complexities of simultaneous longing and denial. It is precisely the proximity to danger, the lure of prohibition, the seamy side of

shame that creates the heat that draws us toward our desires, and that makes desire and pleasure so resistant to rational explanation. It is also what makes pleasure, not a contradiction of or haven from danger, but rather a close relation. These aspects of desire have been marginalized, if not vanquished, from feminist legal theorizing about women's sexuality.

(2001, p. 207)

They have also been written out of contemporary debates over, and proposed policy solutions to, sexual assault on college campuses.

To be sure, universities have a dismal record of handling intra-student sexual violence, and both state and federal governments have been requiring universities to adopt new policies in the name of improved student safety. In 2014, for example, California passed a law requiring all colleges and universities that receive state monies to adopt an affirmative consent standard as part of the process of determining whether or not a sexual assault has taken place. New York recently passed a similar bill. California's Senate Bill 967 (2014) defined affirmative consent as:

affirmative, conscious, and voluntary agreement to engage in sexual activity. It is the responsibility of each person involved in the sexual activity to ensure that he or she has the affirmative consent of the other or others to engage in the sexual activity. Lack of protest or resistance does not mean consent, nor does silence mean consent. Affirmative consent must be ongoing throughout a sexual activity and can be revoked at any time. The existence of a dating relationship between the persons involved, or the fact of past sexual relations between them, should never by itself be assumed to be an indicator of consent.

These guidelines might serve to protect universities from state and federal sanctions for being in non-compliance with Title IX. It is less clear if they will actually prevent sexual assault. (See Gentile, this volume, for detailed discussion of Title IX in the context of campus sexual harassment policies.)

For the purposes of the conversation in this volume, what interests me is the contraction (pun intended) of the space or the capacity to think, let alone talk about, the messiness of sex and desire. The assertion that yes—and only yes—means yes goes beyond an earlier feminist formula, no means no, and shifts the burden of proof from the one who said no (whom the law imagines as a woman) to the one who *heard* yes (whom the law imagines as a man). Both formulations (no = no and yes = yes) imagine a clear line between no and yes, positing sex and sexual desire as fully conscious, unambiguous, and on the model of a contract. This is sex for an actuarial imagination. There is no unconscious, no possibility of ambivalence, no risk, and—as a result—nothing remotely sexy.

Legal regimes and risk management are not only monopolizing public conversations about sexuality; they are also, I daresay, narrowing the capacity of young people (and not just young people) to imagine what they might want, try it out with others, make mistakes, and try again. What might women, or anybody, get to want? How big can yes be?

In Volume I of *The History of Sexuality*, Foucault famously cautioned: "We must not think that by saying yes to sex, one says no to power" (1978, p. 157). But, as Franke points out, the inverse is also true: saying no to sex does not necessarily mean saying yes to (women's, the patient's, the student's) empowerment (2001, p. 197). There may be no escape route from power, but Foucault himself argues that "where there is power there is resistance" (1978, p. 95). Resistance is immanent to power, not its outside. One form of resistance is to refuse to speak the language of legal regimes and bureaucratic logics or to return their language on altered terms, to "queer" it. There may well be occasions when we need to turn to the law, in cases of rape and sexual coercion, for example. But, when we do so, what will we say and ask for?

As I have argued with respect to the new policies on "affirmative consent," bureaucratic logics of managing and minimizing injury, on the one hand, and legal regimes of punishing crimes, on the other, short-circuit richer, more difficult, and urgently necessary conversations about the life of desire.[4] In short: We (often) fail each other, sometimes profoundly. Our embodied lives with others can thus be sources of joy and also of deep wounding—and sometimes even a little bit of both. But our wounds are not necessarily crime sites, in some strict legal sense. How do we talk about sexual error without falling into hard and fast moral judgments? How can psychoanalysis help us? Can it? With and also against Foucault, I believe it can. (This may be a case of supreme greediness on my part: I want my Foucault, I want my Freud, and I want my queer feminism, too.)

To do so, psychoanalysis will need to disrupt some of its own habituated ways of "thinking sex," to quote the title of Gayle Rubin's (1992) influential essay—which was first given as a talk at the 1982 Barnard Sexuality conference. What habits of thought might psychoanalysis need to reconsider? For one: why is sex the privileged thing analysts must not do with their patients (and professors must not do with their students)? If sex is the privileged thing analyst and patient should not do together, is this due to something inherent in sex or (and) is it rather dynamically produced through the cultural and psychic meanings loaded upon sexual relations, the way sex comes to stand in for and block from view a host of other scary, pleasurable, life-threatening, and life-preserving things people already do or might do with each other? It may well be that psychoanalysis poses the question "what two people can say to each other if they agree not to have sex." But what about all the other precious and preciously intimate things analysts agree not to do with their patients in order to create the "as-if" (Orna Guralnik, this volume) of clinical space? Do analysts—should analysts—have dinner with a patient? Write *with* a patient, and not just about one? Play in a softball league together? What links the nos, or delinks the yeses, to any of these questions from the great big no—and *know*—demanded of sex?

That sex has been the privileged and constructed site for "discovering" and "speaking" the truth of the self in western modernity has become something of its own truism in the wake of Foucault (1978). With Foucault, we have also learned how psychoanalysis has historically been a key site for disciplining and normalizing subjects precisely by encouraging us to identify interiority with sex/uality. And yet, against this disciplinary psychoanalysis, which asks us to replay the primal scene and speak the truth of ourselves by talking about sex, what about the psychoanalysis that encourages rogue selves, fantastic experimentations, creative fictions? This version of psychoanalysis might even open up spaces of freedom, novel modes of becoming, of pleasure, of care, and of relating to self and others. This is psychoanalysis not as the will to knowledge but as the risk—undertaken in company—to un-know who you thought you had to be. Such a psychoanalysis overlaps with Foucault's description of the life stakes of writing: "one writes in order to become other than what one is" (quoted in Halperin, 1995, p. 62). Perhaps the writings in this volume, and the essay by Dimen that inspired them, are part of enabling psychoanalysis to become other than what it has been.

Notes

1 In the new customer-driven, neo-liberal university, this traditional distinction and its power flows may be changing. Websites such as RateMy-Professor.com have also upended conventional notions of who grades whom. Untenured and, especially, adjunct faculty who are hired by the course may be vulnerable to student evaluations of their teaching and, especially, of their assessment practices. A teacher with a reputation for being a hard grader may get lower evaluations and, thus, be at risk of losing her job. I want to be clear that I am not pining for the good old days of the authoritative professor—good old days that were not so good for faculty members (or students, for that matter) who were women, people of color, non-Christian, and/or LGBT. But it is necessary to mark, so to speak, how the corporate re-structuring of the university, whether private or public, is also changing what the experiences and expectations of teaching and being taught feel like.

2 See Levin, 2014 on toughening up and "the persistence of a certain kind of transference toward the candidate" (p. 179) in the training system of psychoanalytic institutes.

3 Calling it *marriage* may be. Anyone who has been in a university long enough, whether as student or professor, has met or at least heard of the tenured professor whose wife was his former student, whether undergraduate or graduate (and it is almost always tenured male professor, female student turned spouse). Heterosexual marriage rehabilitates what might otherwise be seen by some as a boundary violation or lapse in professional judgment. Recognized and sanctioned, by the state no less, their classroom affair would not ordinarily be considered "sexual harassment." Marriage may also come to provide similar alibis for same-sex couples composed of a professor and her/his former student. Prior to the advent of legally recognized same-sex marriage, in some university systems, it has been possible for some same-sex teacher-student couples to receive some form of protection from charges of sexual harassment (against the professor) if the professor notified designated administrative officers at her university about the relationship with a former student

and withdrew from any professional oversight of the student (Wolf and Dolan, 1997). The word "former" is important here. Even in cases where a relationship has been, as it were, indemnified through marriage or (other) bureaucratic regulation, it would be considered unprofessional for a faculty member to continue to teach, advise, or in any way officially mentor his or her spouse. The spouse would be seen as receiving pedagogic and professional advantages—favoritism—not available to other students. Why sexual relations are imagined to disrupt pedagogy and confer unfair pedagogic advantages—as opposed to, say, the advantages that come from being the teacher's cherished non-sexual pet—is never fully spelled out in university policies governing consensual sexual relations between faculty and students (Gallop, 1999). It is just taken for granted that they do. The obviousness of this assumption concerning sexual advantages may be linked to its inverse: sexual violation as the worst imaginable form of injury.

4 For a sobering account of the bureaucratic management of "campus sex" in the neo-liberal university, as well as the psychic space the new campus security regimes are producing and regulating, see Doyle, 2015.

References

Dimen, M. (1984). Politically correct? Politically incorrect? In: C. Vance (Ed.) *Pleasure and danger: Exploring female sexuality.* New York: Pandora Press, 1992, pp. 138–148. Reprint, pp ….

Dimen, M. (2011a). *Lapsus linguae,* or a slip of the tongue? A sexual violation in an analytic treatment and its personal and theoretical aftermath. *Contemporary Psychoanalysis,* 47(1): 35–79.

Dimen, M. (Ed.). (2011b). *With culture in mind: Psychoanalytic stories.* New York: Routledge.

Doyle, J. (2015). *Campus sex, campus security.* Cambridge: Semiotext(e)/ Intervention Series.

Foucualt, M. (1976). *La volonté de savoir.* Paris: Gallimard.

Foucault, M. (1978). *History of sexuality, volume I: An introduction.* Trans. Robert Hurley. New York: Vintage Books.

Foucault, M. (1979). *Discipline and punish: The birth of the prison.* Trans. Alan Sheridan. New York: Vintage Books.

Franke, K. (2001). Theorizing yes: An essay on feminism, law, and desire. *Columbia Law Review,* 101(1): 181–208.

Gallop, J. (1997). *Feminist accused of sexual harassment.* Durham: Duke University Press.

Gallop, J. (1999). Resisting reasonableness. *Critical Inquiry,* 25(3) (Spring): 599–609.

Gentile, K. (2021). When the cat guards the canary: Using bystander intervention towards community-based response. *This volume* (pp. 77–99).

Guralnik, O. (2011). Oedipus, incest and us. IARPP-Colloquium series, No. 18, May 9, 2011 to May 22, 2011. Topic: Muriel Dimen's "*Lapsus linguae,* or a slip of the tongue. Moderators, Katie Gentile and Eyal Rozmarin. Posted 11 May.

Halperin, D.M. (1995). *Saint foucault: Toward a gay hagiography.* Oxford: Oxford University Press.

Kipnis, L. (2015). Sexual paranoia strikes academe. *Chronicle of Higher Education.* 27 Feb. Online edition: http://m.chronicle.com/article/Sexual-Paranoia-Strikes/190351/. Accessed 23 June 2015.

Levin, C. (2014). Trauma as a way of life in a psychoanalytic institute. In: R. Deutsch (Ed.) *Traumatic ruptures: Abandonment and betrayal in the analytic relationship.* New York: Routledge, pp. 176–196.

Pellegrini, A. (1999). Pedagogy's turn: Observations on students, teachers, and transference-love. *Critical Inquiry*, 25(3): 617–625.

Phillips, A. (2002). Introduction. In: *Wild analysis.* London: Penguin Books, pp. vii–xxv.

Phillips, A. (2008). On a more impersonal note. In: L. Bersani and A. Phillips *Intimacies.* Chicago: University of Chicago Press, pp. 89–117.

Rubin, G. (1992). Thinking sex: Notes for a radical theory of the politics of sexuality. In: H. Abelove, M.A. Barale and D.M. Halperin (Eds.) *The lesbian and gay studies reader.* New York: Routledge, pp. 3–44.

Senate Bill 967. 2014. California legislative information. Full text available at: https://leginfo.legislature.ca.gov/faces/billNavClient.xhtml?bill_id=201320140SB967. Accessed 23 May 2015.

Vance, C. (Ed.). (1984). *Pleasure and danger: Exploring female sexuality.* New York: Pandora Press. 1992. Reprint.

Winnicott, D.W. (1965). Communicating and not communicating leading to a study of certain opposites. In: *The maturational processes and the facilitating environment: Studies in the theory of emotional development.* London: The Hogarth Press and the Institute of Psycho-Analysis, pp. 179–192.

Wolf, S. and Dolan, J. (1997). Consenting to relations: The personal pleasures of 'power disparity' in lesbian student-teacher partnerships. In: B. Mintz and E.D. Rothblum (Eds.) *Lesbians in academia: Degrees of freedom.* New York: Routledge, pp. 192–198.

Chapter 10

Boundary trouble in the psychoanalytic republic

Reflections on Muriel Dimen's concept of the primal crime

Charles Levin

The narcissism of the law

There is a theory about the constitution of political power in the European nation state which goes something like this: national sovereignty is a modern concept that extends the principle of the divine right of kings into the secular, quasi-democratic realm of the modern political process. Essentially, this means that the state proposes itself to its people as the foundation of the law under which they live; but in order to do this, it holds in reserve a dimension of "sovereignty" that is in certain respects above the law or outside the law and thus invulnerable to any questioning under the rule of law. Sovereignty is the unproven axiom upon which the system of law rests. It allows the state not only to create exceptions to the law, but to be itself a supreme exception. This tacit "contract" provides the semantic and rhetorical basis for common political phrases like "for reasons of state," and "national security." The discourse founded in this notion of sovereignty provides the largely unexamined but still very effective rationale for national governments to operate outside constitutional law, even as they claim to represent it.[1]

Psychoanalysis as an institution and as professional practice was established culturally in a manner analogous to this modern discourse of political and social authority as grounded in "sovereignty." Freud (1912b) described the social dynamic very well in *Totem and Taboo*: he suggested that social order was grounded in the ritualized recollection and expiation of a crime—the murder of the primal father—in such a way that the crime itself becomes the foundation of the law. One might say that in Freud's Hobbesian version of the state of nature, the unbridled "sovereignty" of the primitive father of the "primal horde" represented a kind of idealized lawlessness. But unlike Hobbes, Freud's conception of this original state was not an abstract "war of all against all"—it was already quite explicitly social and familial in its emphasis on the sovereignty vested in the person of the primitive, pre-social "father." (*Jus primae noctis* is just one example of how this idealized state of lawlessness can be institutionalized under the very systems of law that supposedly overthrew it.) For Freud, it was this sovereign power—the primordial sexual narcissism of the primal father—that the patricidal brotherhood transmuted into the force of the law, establishing a more equitable social order, or what we now conceptualize as the sovereignty of the nation state—the contemporary form of patriarchy. Freud commented elsewhere that his study of totemism "leads direct to the origins of the most important institutions of our civilization, of the structure of the state, of morality and religion, and, moreover, of the prohibition against incest and conscience" (1914, p. 37). It also throws light on the foundations of the psychoanalytic order itself.

The political theory of sovereignty also suggests an analogue of Freud's metapsychological discourse on sexuality, notably his writings on instinctual life up to 1914. As we see in the concept of the primal father, Freud's idea was essentially that sexuality is constitutive of the individual and social order while remaining the one element that functions independently of that order. The power of this thing (or force) lies in the fact that it is kept hidden, or in some other way mitigated, by the social forms that it "drives." There is also a connection to the modern concept of the incest taboo, as exemplified in Freud's oedipal theory of the "nuclear complex," and Levi-Strauss's (1949) idea that the prohibition of incest marks the liminal, undecidable, ultimately unintelligible boundary between nature and culture—once again, the paradoxical "sovereignty" of sexuality in its self-limiting creation of the "law."

From this perspective, Muriel Dimen's proposal to revisit psychoanalytic ethics in the light of her own experience of a sexual boundary violation opens up a new dimension of reflection for clinical psychoanalysis. Drawing on the painful evolution of her own professional consciousness over four decades, Dimen showed not only that psychoanalysis remains blind to the social implications of its own theories, but that it needs to take in a strong dose of these theories if it wishes to thrive. By metaphorically "flipping the couch" (Dimen 2011, p. 52), her work has had the effect of liberating the repressed analytic unconscious: a new discursive energy, previously tied down by vigorous professional defences, has been released.

In the classical model, the release of repressed energy through analytic work often translates into a heightening of negative transference (Fernando 2010). This phenomenon is also observable in the social arena of psychoanalysis. Our traditional silence and hypocrisy about sexual misconduct represent our unanalyzed collective negative transference to the profession itself. When the problem is forced to our attention, typically through scandal, this emerges as barely contained hostility, especially toward "whistleblowers," often patients. As Dimen (2011) has described, analysts who have been patients exposed to boundary violations are faced with enormous emotional hurdles—it is extremely difficult and professionally dangerous to speak out (see also Burka 2008, 2014; Dimen 2014; Sundelson 2003; Wallace 2007; Young 2014). Paradoxically, the boundary violators themselves can also be thought of as victims of displaced negativity arising from the undoing of repression, if only because their transgressions are experienced by the community as accusations against all of us (Dimen 2016). At the collective level, sexual boundary violations act like unwelcome interpretations of our unconscious professional life and our collective sense of guilt. As we have struggled with these over the past three or four decades (not longer), we have gradually come to recognize the need for a searching reconceptualization of the psychoanalytic profession along cultural and social lines.

As I read her, Dimen is suggesting that we have been practicing in a kind of ethical abyss of unresolved transference to ourselves as a group. The problem can also be conceived in terms of Winnicott's (1974) "fear of breakdown" (Levin 2016). Like any individual, the psychoanalytic group unconscious is inhabited by "hidden observers" who have been actively repressed or dissociated (Levin 2010). To grasp this we need to think of the individual analytic practitioner as a corporate entity. Indeed, our "training" philosophies implicitly set out to achieve characterological assimilation to a collective stereotype. For this reason among others, the traumatic rigors of analytic training easily slip into a transgenerational dynamic (Levin 2014). Emboldened by a fantasy about ourselves as "specialists of mental suffering," we submit to a punishing regime that forges our identity as analysts in the reified image of uncanny, haunted qualities whose origins we misrecognize. The idealized asceticism of this pedagogical model has potentially constructive but also inevitably destructive consequences.

The closing of the psychoanalytic mind

The specific action of psychoanalysis, as Freud insisted in the early years of its evolution, was connected to the proposition that psychoanalysis created special conditions under which social taboos, generally the various prohibitions on sexual thoughts and feelings, could be safely transgressed in the protective company of another. More precisely, the aim of psychoanalysis, as Freud first conceived it, was to think the unthinkable and/or to remember the unrememberable—specifically, *incest*. For this reason, he never located the sources of "resistance" to psychoanalytic investigation exclusively in the individual patient. As the Dora case illustrates, Freud understood—and soon came to understand even more—that in his work with individual patients, he was asking them not only to suspend their allegiance to certain fundamental social norms, but to abandon unconscious identifications with powerful authority figures, notably the father (Freud 1912a, p. 101). It was in this sense that psychoanalysis actually originated in what might be described as a *social boundary violation*; it was a deliberate and controversial attempt to defy—even against the wishes of the patient—powerful social taboos on the expression of sexual thinking and behavior.

But of course Freud was ambivalent about this, because the terms of his social rebellion remained entirely within the patriarchal model of relationships. He positioned psychoanalysis in the role of killing the primal father, "the violent and jealous father who keeps all the females for himself and drives away his sons as they grow up" (1912b, p. 141). But then, in his institutional politics, through what he described as "deferred obedience" (p. 143), he reinstated "the dead father who became stronger than the living one" (p. 143). Thus, in its origins, psychoanalysis can fairly be described as inherently ambivalent in its relationship to social authority. As an institution, psychoanalysis became a "totemic religion," which "arose from the filial sense of guilt" (p. 145), but also retained a secretly rebellious mood of "festival," understood as "a permitted, or rather an obligatory, *excess*, a solemn breach of a prohibition" (p. 140, emphasis added).

This inherent ambivalence about authority makes psychoanalysis uncomfortable in its own skin. There has always been an element of malaise haunting its official existence. In recent decades, we have become much more aware that this uneasiness is related to the troubled political history of the discipline. When, while ridiculing Jung and Adler, Freud explained the need to create "some headquarters whose business it would be to declare: 'All this nonsense is nothing to do with psychoanalysis'" (Freud 1914, p. 43), he set in motion the repressive dynamics of sovereign power.

The whole point of psychoanalysis was to question the objectivity of culturally received boundaries and categories, to demonstrate the complicity of various energies and areas of life that would normally have been segregated in Freud's day. Yet Freud's call for an authority to protect his ideas about infantile sexuality and the unconscious would become the basis for their practical negation through conservative institutionalization. To save Freud's inspiration, the International Psychoanalytic Association became its tomb. Bion (1970, esp. pp. 75–82) described this dynamic of the psychoanalytic "Establishment" when he reflected on the dialectical relationship between "the mystic and the group." Psychoanalysis set itself up as the "exception that proves the rule" of the sexual unconscious; it began to imagine itself as an entity existing outside and above sexuality and the unconscious—"conflict free"—in order to establish the legitimacy of its power and its right to govern a certain epistemological, but also clinical territory.

Of course, though we are the heirs of Freud, we can be forgiven if we remain equivocal about sexuality. It is a hard subject to debate openly and realistically in public—especially difficult for professionals who depend upon the public trust for their living. After all, psychoanalysts are licensed to "tinker" with people's minds. For this and a variety of other reasons, in clinical theory, we tend to downplay the theoretical importance of the sexual, often by treating it as a mere secondary construct, like a symptom, a defense, or a cultural variation, rather than as a primary elemental force, a deep-seated psychological motive, or (as Freud thought) the originary source of psychopathology. Even those among us who maintain Freud's dictum of the primacy of the sexual tend to do so, in the manner of Laplanche (2015), by cleansing sexuality of biological connotations and exempting adult sexual behavior as irrelevant to psychoanalysis—we claim that it is only "infantile sexuality" that needs to be analysed. But how to distinguish between adult and infantile sexuality? In a most interesting discussion, Meltzer (1973) insisted on the difference between "the polymorphous nature of adult sexuality," which is none of the analyst's business, in contrast to "infantile and perverse elements in our patient's material" (p. 72), which need to be analysed. But after assuring us that "what is adult and private is of no analytic concern," Meltzer then admits that we really have very little idea what we are doing in this regard: "analytic theory has not yet made clear the parameters of adult sexuality so that its richly polymorphous nature can be surely distinguished from the proliferating polymorphism and perversity of infantile sexuality" (p. 65).

If such an important distinction cannot be maintained in practice, might this disqualify psychoanalytic treatment as simply too "dangerous" a method? Or conversely, if the distinction can be sustained, would it not muddy the waters when the question of sex between patient and analyst arises? In fact, a transgressing analyst, possibly even in contradiction with his own published statements about the elusiveness of unconscious mental processes, might well resort to such a distinction in defense of his unethical actions. Such an analyst might argue in a court of law that the patient was a Ph.D in psychology, well-versed in the concept of transference; and that sexual relations with her were part of an adult consensual relationship and therefore not a breach of psychoanalytic ethics. In fact, statements like this have been made even when sexual relations continued during the analysis and the patient was still paying the analytic fee.

Writing of the relation between the psychoanalytic "Mystic" and the psychoanalytic "Establishment," Bion (1970) sagely proposed that

> [t]he individual ... must be able to distinguish between himself
> as an ordinary person and his view that he is omniscient and
> omnipotent. It is a step towards recognition of a distinction

between the group as it really is and its idealization as an embodiment of the omnipotence of the individuals who compose it. Sometimes the separation fails and the group is not only seen to be ideally omnipotent and omniscient but believed to be so in actuality.

(p. 76)

When there is an egregious boundary violation and the profession is caught with its pants down, we tend to fall back on our idealization of ourselves as a group with special knowledge and powers, and to segregate the individual who contradicts this (Dimen 2016; Gabbard 2016; Levin 2016). Sexuality suddenly and magically becomes something relatively simple and straightforward that we understand very well—a practical thing that we are able to control by means of ethical rules and education. SBV may be tricky to define—that we will admit; but like pornography, "we know it when we see it" (Greenberg 2008, p. 889). Quite rightly, in this context, but also in order to cleanse ourselves, we try to delegitimize any appeal to the ambiguity of sexuality as a mitigating factor in instances of patient-analyst sexual relations. We counter that this inherent ambiguity—the elusiveness of the unconscious and the complexity of infantile sexuality—is precisely what necessitates adherence to the rule of abstinence.

That the occurrence of SBV needs to be identified clearly, despite the fuzziness of the words "sexual" and "boundary," does not free us from the nagging sense that the analytic profession has tangled itself up in a significant discrepancy. On the subject of the primal crime, we have been cultivating a serious blind-spot.

Cultural origins of the psychoanalytic republic: Plato

Historically, the inherent omnipotence of analytic institutes created an atmosphere of exceptionalism with regard to the sexual unconscious of its members. Training analysts married their patients and even psychopaths were tolerated and covered up for as long as the institute in question could get away with it. This contradiction is not accidental. It is a deep-seated cultural pattern characteristic of patriarchal groups organized around a hermetic "training" mythology: the sense of privilege is usually couched in an ethos of idealized asceticism, whether it be that of the celibate priest, the Buddhist master, or the training analyst.

The irony is that psychoanalysis began as an opportunity to think about incest, already a risqué proposition; yet it also offers an exquisite opportunity to act it out. In either case, psychoanalysis provides a practical demonstration of the way in which the atmosphere of incest (one might say its conative dimension) migrates throughout the infinite network of human relationships. If one accepts this clinical observation (we might now redescribe it broadly as a consequence of human narcissism, rather than just sexuality per se), it is easier to appreciate Freud's tendency to encourage an ethos of ascetic rationalism, as summarized in the holy trinity of the classical analytic stance: anonymity, abstinence, and neutrality. Freud not only wanted to protect himself from emotional storms (for example by sitting out of view); he foresaw the legitimate need for the analyst, in the service of the patient, to contain and withstand the pressure of powerful unconscious movements, the affective drifts gathering, and getting trapped in, his consulting room.

There is a striking affinity between this rationalist ethos and the dominant trends in classical Western thought. Freud has been pictured in various ways—as the solitary figure in a Caspar David Friedrich landscape, an emblem of the Kantian sublime, steadfastly observant in the face of overpowering nature; or as the Socratic advocate of an ideally ordered Republic, recognizing the psychic reality of oceanic feelings, while banishing the musicians and artists.

The connection to Plato is not just a matter of spinning psychoanalytic ideas one way or another, as Romantic, Aristotelian, or Positivist: there is a root relationship to Plato at the level of institutional vision and educational order. Like celibacy in the service of God and traditional seminary education, psychoanalytic training closely resembles Plato's educational program for the Republic, and its grooming of the ruling class of "philosopher kings." Conceived originally in the ad hoc form of educational outreach, with discretionary powers to recruit new analysts wherever they could be found (Leffert 2010, Ch. 7), institute practices evolved in the 1930s into *de facto* seats of psychoanalytic power, in the style of Plato's "Rulers." Applicants for psychoanalytic training were and still are judged on the impressionistic evaluation of their "character" (usually based on three separate one hour interviews)—not just their academic merits. Procedures like this may be common in the business world and post-graduate education, but psychoanalytic institutes actually believed in their clinical objectivity. As is still suggested on the IPA (2007) website page on training models, "pluralism and democracy have become buzz words for anything goes ... democracy has certain limits in a psychoanalytic society."

The conventional rationale for this character-based procedure was that psychoanalysis had a sacred trust (beyond politics, as Plato claimed for his ruling elite) to serve the best interests of the clinical population by making a very careful selection of only the most gifted, but also the most upright and respectable character types (see for example Britton 2003). Part of this pedagogical storyline has to do with a judgment about whether a person who wants to become an analyst is "analyzable." Emphasizing the need for a good experience of personal analysis, this would seem on the surface to make eminent sense: analysts themselves need analysis, and we cannot really pretend to analyze others without having been analyzed ourselves. The giveaway lies in the falsely objectivistic form of the language. We do not say that a person has had an experience of analysis—we say that he/she has been "analyzed"— by a *training analyst*. The reality in practice is that applicants were and often still are screened according to a normative model of compliant character traits, suiting them for a psychologically brutal regimen of "training."

The educational assumption (not unfounded) is that there is something counter-intuitive and even unnatural, if not slightly inhumane, about the psychoanalytic treatment procedure. The joke making the rounds among candidates and supervisors alike is always: "Don't just do something, sit there!" This quip captures the inherently tension-ridden technical and emotional difficulties of doing effective open-ended, non-directive psychotherapy. On this basis, it was easy for analytic institutes, falling back on the tradition of strict medical hierarchy, to overlook unjust uses of authority and to exaggerate the pedagogical value of stress as a goad to transform the personalities of trainees, if not to break their spirit: after all, they were going to have to do what does not naturally come to them. Like its not so distant cousin, military training, analytic training holds that in order to make a good psychoanalytic soldier, there has to be, as Plato (1987, p. 245) recommended for philosopher kings, a "turning around of the mind." Plato added that turning the mind around "might be made a subject of professional skill."

Like conventional analytic arguments about the nature of the analyst's special skill—that it is a uniquely instilled capacity to screen out incidentals in order to make contact with the unconscious—Plato explained that, in the education of the philosopher, "the mind must be turned away from the world of change until its eye can bear to look straight at reality." Of course, there is a difference between Plato's and Freud's metaphors of the reality that one has to be trained to look straight at. Plato's exhortation to learn how to stare directly into the blinding sunlight of truth is conceptually more straightforward than Freud's idiosyncratic explanation to Lou Salomé: "I have to blind myself artificially in order to focus all the light on one dark spot, renouncing cohesion, harmony, rhetoric, and everything which you call symbolic, frightened as I am by the experience" (1916, p. 45). According to Grotstein (2007, p. 1), Bion rephrased Freud's formulation as follows: "when conducting an analysis, one must cast a *beam of intense darkness* so that something which has hitherto been obscured by the glare of the illumination can glitter all the more in the darkness."

Psychoanalysis seems a far cry from Plato's image of escaping the dark cave of illusions and getting used to the light of the sun. As psychoanalysts, we clearly want to get back into the cave where it seems we have left something important behind, illusion or flickering shadow though it may be, something of singular rather than generic value that is not simply washed out in the solar blanching of "Truth." Yet the underlying structure of the arguments, the special pleading in favor of an authoritarian induction of optimally preconceived states of mind, is very similar after two and a half millennia.

Cultural origins of the psychoanalytic republic: Moses and the submissive transformation of narcissism

The harshness and unrealistic asceticism of psychoanalytic institutional culture derives not from psychoanalytic principles but from traditional patriarchal forms; they contribute to a dangerous underlying combination of feelings: biting deprivation sharpened by a sense of entitlement. The implicit claim to have transcended the sexual unconscious through rigorous training encourages its return in professionally inappropriate ways, including defiant acting out against psychoanalysis itself (Celenza 2007; Saketopoulou, this volume). Since roughly 1980, we have been awakened through public concern over the exploitation of power differentials in professional helping relationships, typically the male analyst and female patient (Gabbard 1989). But there is a sense in which the plight of the patient-victim remains, in the imaginary of organized psychoanalysis, merely a form of "collateral damage" (Burka 2008; Sundelson 2003; Wallace 2010; Young 2014), almost incidental from the institutional point of view. One does not hear about psychoanalytic groups making direct reparation to patients sexually exploited by one of their members.

Specific to this dynamic is the socially privileged violence of the father-son relationship, and the secret pleasure that each takes vicariously in the hidden advantages of the other's position. The drama of their relationship displaces attention away from those who have been used up in their mutual struggle, such as the victims of sexual misconduct by analysts. Between symbolic father and symbolic son, there is a kind of secret understanding that thrives, as I shall argue, through a particular form of projective identification, the submissive transformation of narcissism.[2] As we see reflected in the theoretical literature on projective identification, the object of this defensive process leaps like a quantum electron from one sphere to another, from the world of internal objects to actual persons, the group, and back. This violent reciprocity locks in the participants and mesmerizes the surrounding social group through the inception of a vicious circle that transforms any critique of the father into a re-enactment of his authority—as Freud brilliantly described in *Totem and Taboo*. Smith (2008) has observed:

> [I]f punishment is *simultaneously* punishment of self and of others, it creates its own vicious circle, with punishment of others requiring punishment of self (because of guilt) and punishment of self requiring punishment of others (because of envy). Thus the vicious circle is set in motion …
>
> (p. 208)

The predominance of this dynamic within the group both produces and presupposes the marginalization of women, not only as sexual and affectionate objects to be fought over and exchanged (Levi-Strauss 1949; Rubin 1975), but in their implicitly assigned role as paralyzed witnesses of the narcissistic struggle for male succession: the Law of the Father and Son.

For Freud (1921, p. 105f.), primary infantile identifications are always with the father. He was a keen observer of patriarchal psychology (Mitchell 1974) and fascinated by the father-son relationship. The historical figures he most admired were all patriarchal rebels, even regicides, who embodied qualities from all sides of the equation, being very good at defying masculine authority, but also excellent at imposing it. There is a distinctly undemocratic strain in Freud's choice of heroes, such as Hannibal and Cromwell.

Moses was perhaps his favorite. Freud was convinced that the spiritual liberator of the Jewish people was in fact the son of an Egyptian pharaoh, an idea which, as Edward Said (2004) has pointed out, expresses "in our age of vast population transfers, of refugees, expatriates and immigrants ... the diasporic, wandering, unresolved cosmopolitan consciousness of someone who is both inside and outside his or her community" (p. 53). We know that Freud dreaded the prospect of psychoanalysis becoming a "Jewish science;" yet, as Aron and Starr (2013) have argued, psychoanalysis might more appropriately be described as a nomadic, hybrid, "optimally marginal" enterprise without any true "headquarters": "Only someone immersed in the culture yet not subsumed by it is in a position to offer the kind of critique that psychoanalysis offers" (Aron & Starr, p. 240).

Unfortunately, the story of Moses in the Old Testament is not only about liberation and traveling, but also the establishment of an absolute, centralized and unforgiving authority (which Freud admiringly described as monotheism). In a style of argument reminiscent of the modern theory of the state, and Freud's anthropological speculations, Exodus (n.d.) sets out to rationalize and glorify the institution of sovereign power, a state of exception, through a mythic invention about return from exile and the (re-)establishment of a homeland. However, the maternal part of "home" is almost entirely occluded. Everything is about the negotiation between the father and the son. In explicit detail, *Exodus* recounts the drama of Moses' omnipotent delusions of grandeur, his bloody suppression of his own people, and the destruction of their creativity and freedom. Like Abraham before him, Moses is torn between the love of his people, his children (his love for them and theirs for him) and his murderous but also frightened impulse to slaughter and punish them, to assert his will over the "anarchy" of the group—in other words, the threat posed to his authority by the emergence of separate centers of intentionality and initiative.

It is interesting that the figure of Moses simultaneously represents many different positions within the father-son constellation: successful rebellion against the oppressive and murderous father (the Pharoah), abject submission to and loyalty to that same father (Yahweh—the Lord), and the oppressive and murderous father himself. This way of rolling everything together into one (obedient son, rebellious son, beloved father, and murderous father) contributes to the cultural privilege of the father-son relationship. Its protean dominance suggests a social climate organized through projective identification along sadomasochistic lines, a syndrome brilliantly described by Benjamin (2004) as the relational impasse of reversible complementarity in which doer and done-to endlessly trade positions and eviscerate awareness of anything outside their privileged coupling.

It is psychologically possible for Moses to represent both father and son, savior and killer, because he and his social group are in a state of dissociation in which they have displaced responsibility for everybody's narcissism onto a fictional entity, the "dead father" as symbolized by the god of the Old Testament.[3] The underlying social madness of this situation is contained within the group through submission to this irrational god, but the latter requires acting out through sacrifice. It is not an accident that Christ's destruction and resurrection are described as a "passion." In *Exodus*, the tribes of Israel are mesmerized and confused by their omnipotent patriarch's struggle with his own demons. Moses' relationship with the disembodied voice of Jawheh is mysterious, erotic and narcissistically thrilling. There are burning bushes. When Moses returns to his people from Mount Sinai, where Yahweh has been penetrating his ear for forty days and nights, we find him in a state of agitated excitement, visibly flushed.

What immediately follows is Moses' famous outburst of rage against his people. It is important to remember the nature of the gift that he is bearing on his return from the Mount. He has not only the Ten Commandments in hand, but also Yahweh's meticulous, intricate, and aesthetically detailed instructions for the creation of the Tabernacle. The psychic content of these gifts is very precious to Moses personally, something like the solution to his (and our own) deepest turmoil. Indeed, the gifts contain an elaborate program for the institutionalization and control of the most primitive aspects of human narcissism. The architectural instructions for the Tabernacle suggest implicitly what the commandments directly state: human narcissism will be embodied in an extraordinary collective fantasy of unlimited power and glory, projected into a forbidding father figure who regularly exhibits attitudes of omnipotence, exclusivity, entitlement, superiority, vanity, cruelty, vengefulness, jealousy and envy. If this solution can be accepted and tolerated by the group, then everyone can expect to feel both exonerated, protected, and well-compensated for allegiance to the new social order, while still enjoying, at least vicariously, the selfishness and self-interest that have been partially (or in the case of women, almost wholly) renounced through this collective form of projective identification, the submissive transformation of narcissism.

The first commandment, announcing the monotheistic creed that so impressed Freud, brings the news that the Lord on the Mount is the one and only true god: "You shall have no other gods before me," Moses says on his behalf (*Exodus* 20, 3). In case of any doubt about the absoluteness of this principle, the second commandment lays out the narrow range of options left open for the Lord's subjects:

> You shall not make for yourselves an idol [graven image], nor any image [likeness] of anything that is in the heavens above, or that is in the earth beneath, or that is in the water under the earth: you shall not bow yourself down to them, nor serve them, for I, Yahweh [the Lord] your God, am a jealous God, visiting the iniquity of the fathers on the children, on the third and on the fourth generation of those who hate me, and

showing lovingkindness [mercy] to thousands of those who love
me and keep my commandments.

(Exodus 20, 4–6)

Not only does this commandment forbid making images of the
Lord without his permission, it forbids the making of any image of
any kind—"any likeness of *any thing*." It is not just that the Lord's
subjects might think of worshipping something other than Him.
They might also be *thinking* of something else—not necessarily
a rival god, but still a being other than Him. They might have
a thought and try to represent it, without His permission.

This way of establishing divine rule ties in closely with Platonism.
The Law, like the Platonic Forms, precedes its manifestations and
approximations, and rules independently of them. All unauthorized
"copies" or "imitations" are deemed corrupt and illegitimate and
subject to suppression and severe punishment. In this sense, the
principle of sovereignty can be traced to fantasies about an idealized
state of subjective freedom: it is the rule of absolute narcissism as
vicariously lived out by the human subjects who submit themselves
to it: sovereignty is complete and self-sufficient, including exclusive
copyright on everything in the universe.

The ban on independent communication codified in the second
commandment addresses a very important issue from the point of
view of social control. It is not just the nasty side of narcissism, the
violent grandiosity, that needs to be shut down and reorganized. If
there is to be a central authority, then creativity itself, the possibility
that an unauthorized "I" might be capable of initiative, also falls
under deep suspicion—all the more so because, from the point of
view of the patriarch, creativity is much more difficult to harness
than destructiveness; it is inherently subversive of stereotyped
authority, whereas violence easily falls into line with that same
authority. This hatred of independent initiative within the group is
reinforced in the third and fourth commandments. Only in the fifth
commandment does the decalogue turn to the question of how
people should treat each other. This two-tiered structure creates
a moral vicious circle, in which the stifling of independent initiative
in the first four commandments (only me, no independent creativity,
no criticism, compulsory day of worship) creates a motive for the

interpersonal crimes proscribed in the last six (treat your parents as you would Me, no killing, no adultery, no stealing, no lying about your neighbors, no coveting your neighbor and his possessions, including his wife, manservant, oxen, etc.). As we have seen, the dynamic relationship between sexual transgression and exaggerated asceticism in psychoanalysis has a similar structure, in which envious attacks on youthful creativity are met with guilty reprisals, and so on, ad infinitum. This is an aspect of the Oedipus story that psychoanalysis has consistently under-represented. Klein (1957, p. 231) saw the vicious cycle of envy as originating in the infant's destructive impulse toward the good object, leading to guilty self-devaluation, which only increases the envy, and therefore the attacks on goodness. Another way to look at this would be that in patriarchal systems, the father's murderous wishes induce a guilty devaluation of loving impulses, resulting in tremendous envy of love (idealized in the mother-infant relationship), and a vicious cycle of narcissistic identifications and reprisals between father and son which chronically undermines the potential for loving relationships in the group as a whole.

The Lord's (our) fear and loathing of initiative brings us to His instructions for the building of the Tabernacle, which leave no doubt that He is indeed the Supreme Architect, not only of the universe, but more importantly of His Own Worship. The exact dimensions, layerings and textural refinements of the space that will sound the Lord's disembodied voice (only to the initiated, who must be wearing the proper garments) are carefully defined, right down to the color of the threads that shall be interwoven and the materials that shall be worked and combined (only by artisans of such and such a type).[4] There is no room here for any person or group to have an idea of their own about how to pay homage to the Lord, how to celebrate His Majesty. In case anyone should miss this point, *Exodus* presents the whole plan in all its detail *twice*, somewhat absurdly: first before Moses' slaughter of the worshippers of the golden calf, and then once again afterwards, for emphasis. They provide a perfect frame for the following dramatic scene:

> When Moses saw that the people had broken loose ... then Moses stood in the gate of the camp, and said, "Whoever is on

Yahweh's side, come to me!" ... Thus says Yahweh, the God of
Israel, 'Every man put his sword on his thigh, and go back and
forth from gate to gate throughout the camp, and everyman kill
his brother, and everyman his companion, and every man his
neighbour.'" The sons of Levi did according to the word of
Moses, and there fell of the people that day about three thousand men. Moses said, "Consecrate yourselves today to
Yahweh, yes, every man against his son, and against his brother,
that he may bestow upon you a blessing this day.

(Exodus 32, 25–29)

Like Plato's *Republic, Exodus* makes very clear what is at stake in
an elite membership group based on arcane knowledge: there is an
inherent risk of structuring power around the concept of exclusive
ownership. The effect can be a kind of social copyright, which
becomes the template for the regulation of behavior and the sup-
pressive molding of subjectivity. The institution demands conformity
to a certain moralistic stereotype—otherwise, one cannot belong.
Psychoanalytic groups provide an example.

The principle of sovereignty extends the biblical conceptions of
power and authority into the realm of secular politics, the division
of labor, and professional identity. One might say that sovereignty is
a generalization of projective identification in the collective form of
submissive transformation of narcissism. It involves an idealized
attribution of socially problematic aspects of narcissism into an
externalized fictional agency—an objectified subject who is imagined
as the author of the group and its protector. From the perspective
of *Totem and Taboo*, the primitive narcissism of the primal father is
idealized in a form that controls the group and binds it together. In
exchange for submission to this absolute but disembodied form of
centralized authority, narcissism in the group can be shaped, externalized when necessary, and generally disavowed, while still being
enjoyed vicariously through its authority to reign upon the group,
and the license it provides certain members of the group to act in
its name, to bully, judge, and even to kill, rape or maim. The affective relish with which otherwise civilized people will observe or
commit torture, and kill those perceived to transgress sovereign
authority, serves both to bind the group to some kind of regularized

order, while at the same time providing a framework for enjoying the impulses which only the one Lord is authorized to enact.

The compliant-transgressive false self

Given the underlying cultural/unconscious conditions of the analytic profession, it becomes possible to conceptualize the continuing presence, and prevalence, of sexual misconduct, as a form (albeit perverse) of truth telling. The sexually transgressing analyst—*ceux qui passe a l'acte* (Urtubey 2006)—expresses not only the sexual wish, but also the forbidden *knowledge* of the group as a whole, in its history and present state. Here we can take another cue from Bion (1963, pp. 45ff): the Eden myth, and the Oedipal dynamic, are not only stories about the consequences of sexual rebellion; they also symbolize the psychic dangers, and profound conflicts, aroused by any serious quest for knowledge, including self-knowledge: "Oedipus represents the triumph of determined curiosity over intimidation" (p. 49). We can make jokes about the transgressing analyst's desire to "know" the patient (in the biblical sense); but there may also be in the scenario of sexual transgression a distorted and desperate form of the wish, expressed through defiance of the psychoanalytic Establishment (Bion 1970), to find a deeper, perhaps even mystical truth, for which the patient may serve as a kind of muse, representing the living embodiment of what it means to know and master the human condition. There is a sense in which all of the most creative analysts, Freud, Jung, Ferenczi, Klein, and Winnicott, to mention only a few, were incestuous and transgressive analysts in this ambiguous and potentially dangerous sense. Of course, as Freud quipped in his rationale for a psychoanalytic "headquarters," "none of this nonsense has anything to do with psychoanalysis." But there it is all the same, and for what it is worth: our collective oedipal phantasy.

The social dynamics of transgression are implicit in the cultural origins of the profession itself. By reframing the ethical problem of psychoanalysis in terms of the "primal crime," Muriel Dimen undercuts our tendency to moralistically indict and excommunicate individual analysts who "transgress." Transgression is no longer a figment of the individual alone, whose secret misconduct is accidentally discovered by the group. Rather, as a corporate entity, the individual transgressor expresses an unconscious problematic of the group.

Dimen's allusion to Freud's speculative anthropology unsettles our professionally self-serving assumptions about the otherness of the unethical in our midst by implying that our analytic rituals are invested in a deeper group logic of sacral repetition and expiation. If analysts' sexual boundary violations represent something "primal," as she suggests, then these crimes cannot be morally extraneous to psychoanalysis; in other words, it would be specious to claim that they are "*un*psychoanalytic"—"not psychoanalysis," as the refrain goes. They must have been present at the origin, somehow implicit in the formation of the psychoanalytic idea, constitutive of the profession.

In effect, Dimen asks us an embarrassing question: how could we fail so massively, and for nearly a century, to be curious about our own sexual behavior? How did we, the descendants of Freud, get ourselves into a position where we would be so surprised by sex? If this line of questioning is valid, then we need to consider the possibility that analysts' sexual misconduct, whatever its particular combination of causes, includes a "return of the repressed," a frustrated expression, albeit perverse and secretive, of an institutional malaise.

On this view, sexual boundary violations are indeed a kind of truth telling, to the extent that they also represent a symptomatic displacement and disavowal of something important about being a psychoanalyst. Sexual transgressions may often be figuring the wish to reverse and re-enact the experience of "traumatic narcissism" (Shaw 2014). The deeper ethical problem for psychoanalysis would then be its failure to recognize that the origins of the analyst's trauma lie not just in the individual analyst's personal history, but also in the history and nature of psychoanalysis itself. The supposition would be that psychoanalysis has failed to settle accounts with the emotional consequences of being a psychoanalyst, including the unconscious residues of psychoanalytic history, as institutionalized in professional hierarchies and transmitted through training procedures. The issue for discussion would be whether and how much the psychoanalytic profession resembles a "relational system of subjugation" (Shaw 2014), rather than a supportive enhancement of a person's capacity for analytic work.

Like any perspective on the unconscious, individual or collective, this way of looking at the problem of sexual misconduct is only as good as its reception in the group, and as the struggle for understanding it occasions. All we can do at this stage is to try to work out its implications.

One of the obvious implications is that we have been hiding something from ourselves. Some indications of this can be found in our use of language, for example the use of the word "boundary." In the last quarter century, psychoanalysis graduated from the militaristic vocabulary of "sexual misconduct" to the technical term "sexual boundary violation," signaling a welcome professional internalization of ethical reasoning, a growing concern with the welfare of the other (Levinas 1998). However there have been complications along the way. "Violation" does a better job than "misconduct" of describing the damaging nature of unethical behavior, but it also feeds into certain professional defenses. The word has a particular connotation that runs counter to the ordinary fuzziness of psychoanalytic concepts; it suggests that psychic phenomena have discrete partitions which can be clearly demarcated and defined. One can see why a crisp word like "boundary" would have appealed in the effort to overcome our profession's resistance to discussing its own ethics in public: it not only cuts through self-serving rationalizations based on psychic ambiguity; it also helps to reassure the public that we do understand the problem and that we have it under control.

But of course what our language conceals from the public, it also conceals from us. Where is the boundary between the individual transgressor and the group to which he or she belongs? Where is the boundary between that group and the abused patient? By assuming the confidence of naming and knowing boundaries, we imagine that we have finished a discussion that has hardly begun.

Perhaps the main reason why it is so difficult to deepen this discussion is that the need for it entails a painful admission. To address the moral complicity of the profession in the individual analyst's transgression is to entertain a whole host of terrible worries that we naturally would prefer not to acknowledge, especially at the level of the threatened group, with all its potential for primitive, regressive emotional violence. It puts us inside Joan Riviere's (1936) shocking description of the depressive position, a desolate place in which, unconsciously, everything seems ruined. As she argued for the individual patient, so for the analytic profession: Efforts at (self-) understanding risk provoking a negative therapeutic reaction. As the individual resists help until the damaged objects can be repaired, so goes the psychoanalytic group. Perhaps we feel that trying to help the profession get better will only make our condition worse, until somehow we find a way to set our damaged progenitors aright.

One of the awful worries that we all live with today in our practice is that perhaps psychoanalysis is actually dead—clinically, culturally, politically, morally. This means that unconsciously or unwittingly we have murdered it—through our hatred and our violations, to be sure, but more importantly, through our failure to acknowledge the social realities of our individual and collective psychic life. This failure is linked to the double bind in Riviere's version of the depressive position. If we don't recognize the "primal crime" as constitutive of psychoanalysis, we are assuming that we are a straightforward technical discipline like any other (as we may imagine the other disciplines), and not an "explosive force," in Bion's description of our predicament (1970, p. 78). If this were true, then we would already be spiritually dead through disaffiliation with our morally ambiguous analytic ancestors. On the other hand, if we had recognized our origins in the "primal crime," this might have meant that psychoanalysis would become so emotionally complicated and unbearable that we would have killed it in the process of trying to live with it.

It is understandable, especially in the present social climate, that we avoid reckoning with the possibility that psychoanalysis is only alive insofar as it remains emotionally in touch with its traumatic birth and childhood, as a devious form of social transgression, involving displaced protest, chronic unrest, and disguised troublemaking. As Wheelis (1958) astutely observed of his own analytic career: "It comes about at times ... that the very conflict which has led one into a certain profession is aggravated by the practice of that profession" (p. 206). The predicament is a real one, which we cannot pretend to resolve through a simple choice to resist or embrace the instrumental technicism of the health industry. In a very real sense, we are trapped by our own history, the circumstances of our cultural self-construction as a field of inquiry, a theory and, whether we like it or not, also a form of treatment.

Whatever we do, we cannot avoid the implication that we are trying to mitigate our guilty sense of participation in the larger social transgression upon which the idea of psychoanalysis was founded. Perhaps this is an aspect of what Muriel Dimen (2011, p. 73) described as "self-shame" ("the condition we dread being found in")—that each sexual scandal in our profession reminds us not only of our own transgressions, or near transgressions, but the shame that we dimly, sometimes keenly, feel—and are made to feel in social concourse—about the bizarre, seemingly even perverse, nature of our work.

Another very painful worry arises from the fact that the characteristics of the malignant narcissistic leader are present in every analyst who sexually abuses a patient, not just the predator type, but also the narcissistically fragile or "lovesick" type (Gabbard & Lester 1995; Celenza & Gabbard 2003) who may be unlikely to repeat the offense. Yet none of us is immune, we have learned to acknowledge, and so in a real sense we all belong to this group (Celenza 2007; Celenza 2014). The profile of the fragile analyst, who may also be prone to "masochistic surrender" (Gabbard & Lester 1995, pp. 113–117), fits with clinical descriptions of the passive compliant narcissist, a common form of "false self syndrome," who is suffering mainly from cumulative trauma and the effects of self-abnegation in formative personal and social relationships.

The idea that submissive narcissism in an adult professional situation might predispose to trauma was actually suggested by Freud in his discussion of the war neuroses. He argued that traumatic reactions can be triggered by a professional conflict between "the soldier's old peaceful ego and his new warlike one" (Freud 1919, p. 209). Freud added (p. 210) "that we have a perfect right to describe repression, which lies at the basis of every neurosis, as a reaction to trauma—as an elementary traumatic neurosis." Connected to the issue of war neurosis, we also know about, but do not really acknowledge, the corrosive effect of working habitually in the position of the helpless witness, which leads to chronic guilt feelings and sometimes pervasive dissociative defenses.

We have often suffered as helpless witnesses in the analytic training process, or in earlier medical education, or psychology internships, where in order to pass muster, to remain in good standing, and to survive the rigors of apprenticeship, we turned a blind eye to injustices inflicted on fellow students, staff, or patients, and ourselves. Historically, we have evinced a curious tolerance for authoritarianism in our midst. If the fragile respectability of the post-Freudian psychoanalytic profession stands for a kind of collective false self, then it may also be that many of us have been thwarted rebels in search of prestigious cover. Further to this institutionalized premium on self-control, the trials of passive witnessing have been built into the corporate identity of the practicing analyst. The general ideal of serving as a resilient container, of learning to preserve the frame even in the face of the patient's desperate "attacks" (the London Kleinians still speak, usually off the record, of "strong" as opposed to "weak" analysts), inevitably places every analyst, of whatever persuasion, in the position of the witness who feels helpless. We may in our practice be temperamentally "active" and "interactive," even eager for "combat" (Hoffman 2009); but we will still wind up feeling trapped in the position of frustrating ineffectuality. Understanding and appreciating the value for the patient of the analyst's quiet receptivity, or unintrusive emotional presence, does not erase the occupational hazard of enduring, day after day, the pressure to renounce one's rescue fantasies (or fantasies of revolt)—to witness suffering without taking direct action to alleviate not only the suffering, but also its impact on oneself.

If we were to consider factors like these in open conversation, we would have to deal with the very likely possibility that the transgression of sexual boundaries is just the "tip of the iceberg." Our ethical problem is much more difficult than that, it would seem, because the analytic situation strips us of conventional narcissistic protections. The professional danger situation is not only sexual desire, which arises intermittently and idiosyncratically, in ways that can usually be identified and handled, but the relentless pressure of ordinary narcissism, and the psychic vulnerabilities it engenders. As Celenza (2020) points out, different kinds of analytic stance may be self-serving for different analytic personality types. Our particular narcissistic susceptibilities are difficult to define publically or to regulate in the impersonal administrative mode. It would appear that the only way we have to handle this level of ethical complexity in a democratic way is through the moral embarrassment—but not shame—of surrendering ourselves to our own method, in some as yet unexplored collective version of the talking cure.

Ordinary people will still—quite literally—back away from us at parties on learning we are psychoanalysts, even in New York, London and Paris. They say something nervously funny about how we might be reading their minds. Naturally, we are dismissive of this stereotyped response to the category "psychoanalyst." But surely it is a reference to a historical reality—the cultural perception of our disguised sexual (but also narcissistic) intrusiveness. Maybe we should respect it more, be more curious about its meaning. If there is still an allergic social response to psychoanalysis, perhaps we should embrace it as a sign of life, if only we could face up to ourselves as a group.

Notes

1 For a stimulating discussion of the sovereignty principle, see Giorgio Agamben (1998). For a contrasting view, see Snyder (2015), who demonstrates that chances of survival for individual Jews in Europe during the period 1933–1945, though always slim, depended crucially on the possession of state citizenship documents, including German ones.
2 Extended discussion of the submissive transformation of narcissism can be found in Giesbrecht and Levin (2012).
3 I refer to the Old Testament rather than the Torah because it was primarily through Christianity that these images of patriarchal privilege and authority were disseminated throughout Western culture.
4 The "orientalism" of the traditional psychoanalytic office décor and the fact that the analyst in the classical position listens and speaks in disembodied, invisible fashion, suggest an objective correlative of the inmost chamber of the Tabernacle, as described in Exodus (n.d.).

References

Agamben, G. (1998). *Homo sacer: Sovereign power and the bare life.* Trans. D. Heller-Roazen. Stanford: Stanford University Press.
Aron, L. & Starr, K. (2013). *A psychotherapy for the people: Toward a progressive psychoanalysis.* New York & London: Routledge.
Benjamin, J. (2004). Beyond doer and done to: An intersubjective view of thirdness. *Psychoanalytic Quarterly* 73 (1): 5–46.
Bion, W.R. (1963). Elements of psycho-analysis. In *Seven servants: Four works by Wilfred R. Bion.* New York: Jason Aronson.

Bion, W.R. (1970). *Attention and interpretation: A scientific approach to insight in psychoanalysis and groups.* London: Tavistock.

Britton, R. (2003). Confidentiality and training analyses. In Levin, et al., ed., *Confidentiality.* pp. 109–112.

Burka, J. (2008). Psychic fallout from breach of confidentiality: A patient/analyst's perspective. *Contemporary Psychoanalysis* 44: 177–198.

Burka, J. (2014). A chorus of difference: Evolving moral outrage to complexity and pluralism. In R. Deutsch ed., *Traumatic ruptures.* pp. 126–143.

Celenza, A. (2007). *Sexual boundary violations: Therapeutic, supervisory and academic contexts.* New York: Jason Aronson.

Celenza, A. (2014). *Erotic revelations: Clinical applications and perverse scenarios.* London and New York: Routledge.

Celenza, A. (2020). Shadows that corrupt: Present absences in the psychoanalytic process. In C. Levin, ed. (2021), *Sexual boundary trouble in psychoanalysis: Clinical perspectives on Muriel Dimen's concept of the 'primal crime'.* London & New York: Routledge.

Celenza, A. & Gabbard, G.O. (2003). Analysts who commit sexual boundary violations: A lost cause? *Journal of the American Psychoanalytic Association* 51: 617–636.

de Urtubey, L. (2006). *Si l'analyste passe a l'acte.* Paris: Presses universitaires de France.

Deutsch, R., ed (2014). *Traumatic ruptures: Abandonment and betrayal in the analytic relationship.* New York and London: Routledge.

Dimen, M. (2011). Lapsus linguae, or a slip of the tongue? A sexual violation in an analytic treatmetn and its personal and theoretical aftermath. *Contemporary Psychoanalysis* 47 (1): 35–79.

Dimen, M. (2014). Foreward: Traumatic ruptures. In R. Deutsch ed., *Traumatic ruptures: Abandonment and betrayal in the analytic relationship.* New York and London: Routledge, pp. xv–xvi.

Dimen, M. (2016). Rotten apples and ambivalence. *Journal of the American Psychoanalytic Association* 64 (2): 361–373.

Exodus. (n.d.). *World English Bible (WEB).*

Fernando, J. (2010). *The processes of defense: Trauma, drives, and reality — A new synthesis.* New York: Aronson.

Freud, S. (1912a). The dynamics of transference. In J. Strachey ed. & Trans., *The standard edition of the psychological works of Sigmund Freud* (vol. 12). London: Hogarth, pp. 99–108.

Freud, S. (1912b). Totem and taboo. In J. Strachey ed. & Trans., *The standard edition of the psychological works of Sigmund Freud* (vol. 13). London: Hogarth, pp. 1–162.

Freud, S. (1914). On the history of the psycho-analytic movement. In J. Strachey ed. & Trans., *The standard edition of the complete psychological works of Sigmund Freud* (vol. 14). London: Hogarth, pp. 7–66.

Freud, S. (1916). Letter from Freud to Lou Andreas Salome, May 25, 1916. *The International Psycho-Analytical Library* 89: 45.

Freud, S. (1919). Introduction to *psycho-analysis and the war neuroses*. In J. Strachey ed. & Trans., *The standard edition of the omplete psychological works of Sigmund Freud* (vol. 17). London: Hogarth, pp. 207–210.

Freud, S. (1921). Group psychology and the analysis of the ego. In J. Strachey ed. & Trans., *The standard edition of the omplete psychological works of Sigmund Freud* (vol. 18). London: Hogarth, pp. 69–143.

Gabbard, G.O., ed (1989). *Sexual exploitation in professional relationships*. Washington, DC: American Psychiatric Press.

Gabbard, G.O. & Lester, E.P. (1995). *Boundaries and boundary violations in psychoanalysis*. New York: Basic.

Giesbrecht, H. & Levin, C. (2012). *Art in the offertorium: Narcissism, psychoanalysis, and cultural metaphysics*. Amsterdam & New York: Rodopi.

Greenberg, J. (2008). Right destination, wrong path. *Psychoanalytic Quarterly* 77: 883–890.

Grotstein, J. (2007). *A beam of intense darkness: Wilfred Bion's legacy to psychoanalysis*. London: Karnac.

Hoffman, I.Z. (2009). Therapeutic passion in the countertransference. *Psychoanalytic Dialogues* 19 (5): 617–637.

IPA. (2007). The three training models. www.ipa.world/IPA/en/Training/3models.aspx

Klein, M. (1957). Envy and gratitude. In *Envy and gratitude & other works: 1946–1963*. New York: Dell, 1975, pp. 176–235.

Laplanche, J. (2015). *The temptation of biology: Freud's theories of sexuality*. Trans. D. Nicholson-Smith. New York: The Unconscious in Translation.

Leffert, M. (2010). *Contemporary psychoanalytic foundations: Postmodernism, complexity, and neuroscience*. London & New York: Rutledge.

Levin, C. (2010). The mind as a complex internal object: Inner estrangement. *Psychoanalytic Quarterly* 79 (1): 95–127.

Levin, C. (2014). Trauma as a way of life in a psychoanalytic institute. In R. Deutsch ed., *Traumatic ruptures: Abandonment and betrayal in the analytic relationship*. London & New York: Routledge, pp. 176–196.

Levin, C. (2016). Fear of breakdown in the psychoanalytic group: Commentary on Dimen. *Journal of the American Psychoanalytic Association* 64 (2): 381–388.

Levin, C., Furlong, A., & O'Neil, M.K., eds (2003). *Confidentiality: Ethical perspectives and clinical dilemmas.* Hillsdale, NJ: The Analytic Press.

Levinas, E. (1998). *Otherwise than being or beyond essence.* Trans. Alphonso Lingis. Pittsburgh, PA: Duquesne University Press.

Levi-Strauss, C. (1949). *The elementary structures of kinship.* New York: Eyre and Spottiswood, 1969.

Meltzer, D. (1973). *Sexual states of mind.* Pertshire, Scotland: Clunie Press.

Mitchell, J. (1974). *Psychoanalysis and feminism.* New York: Vintage.

Plato. (1987). *The republic* (Second Edition). Trans. D. Lee. London: Penguin Classics.

Riviere, J. (1936). A contribution to the analysis of the negative therapeutic reaction. *International Journal of Psycho-Analysis* 17: 304–320.

Rubin, G. (1975). The traffic in women: Notes on the "political economy" of sex. In L. Nicholson ed., *The second wave: A reader in feminist theory.* New York: Routledge, 1997, pp. 27–62.

Said, E. (2004). *Freud and the non-European.* London: Verso.

Saketopoulou, A. (2020). Does the sexual have anything to do with boundary violations? *This volume* (pp. 101–128).

Shaw, D. (2014). *Traumatic narcissism: Relational systems of subjugation.* New York and London: Routledge.

Smith, H.F. (2008). Vicious circles of punishment: A reading of Melanie Klein's *Envy and Gratitude. Psychoanalytic Quarterly* 77: 199–218.

Snyder, T. (2015). *Black earth: The holocaust as history and warning.* New York: Tim Duggan Books.

Sundelson, D. (2003). Outing the victim: Breaches of confidentiality in an ethics procedure. In C. Levin, et al., ed., *Confidentiality.* pp. 184–198.

Wallace, E. (2007). Losing a training analyst for ethical violations: A candidate's perspective. *International Journal of Psychoanalysis* 88: 1275–1288.

Wallace, E. (2010). Collateral damage: Long-term effects of losing a training analyst in ethical violations. *Canadian Journal of Psychoanalysis* 18: 248–254.

Wheelis, A. (1958). *The quest for identity.* New York: Norton.

Winnicott, D.W. (1974). Fear of breakdown. *International Review of Psychoanalysis* 1: 103–107.

Young, C. (2014). Collateral damage: The fallout from analyst loss due to ethical violations. In R. Deutsch ed., *Traumatic ruptures.* pp. 109–125.

Part IV

Psychoanalysis *Unendliche*

Chapter 11

Losing our psychoanalytic virginity

Muriel Dimen and Charles Levin

Introduction

A few months before she died, in preparation for this interview, Muriel Dimen read all the contributions to this book, and also the contributions to its companion volume, *Sexual Boundary Trouble in Psychoanalysis: Clinical Perspectives on Muriel Dimen's Concept of the "Primal Crime,"* including an earlier version of my Introduction, which was written before she became ill. She was pleased with the results and hopeful for our human prospects, if not her own – she knew she was going to die in the very near future.

There is much more that she would have liked to say in response to the material collected in this book, but what she did manage to articulate in those difficult circumstances seems essential to me. Muriel appeared to be indomitable in the face of death, remaining steadfast not only in her faith in the basic goodness of the world, but also able to deal with problems and details that others in her situation would have tossed aside.

I remember an incident with Muriel while crossing the Margit bridge in Budapest, on the way back from a long walk, returning to a conference on Sandor Ferenczi. There was a very large billboard on the Pest side of the Danube. It clashed painfully with the surrounding ambience of stable traditions, the majestic architecture and reassuring semiotics of an historic site, dating from the Austro-Hungarian empire and before.

I commented critically on the billboard – a luridly capitalistic advertisement, probably a lifestyle pitch for a Cola. My objection was that it trivialized the complex historical embeddedness of the place we were in, by claiming revolutionary status for a mediocre product, and fake liberation for those who consume it. Muriel's immediate response was incisive and unforgettable. She said that maybe the co-option of revolutionary messages is inevitable, and that we need to keep an eye on how they nevertheless implicitly carry forward the revolutionary message itself, and the demand for liberation.

The following discussion illustrates Muriel's measured and wise way of thinking about problems like this, with reference to the psychoanalytic profession in particular.

Charles Levin

Dr. Dimen, most readers will be well aware of the depth of your critical analysis of the psychoanalytic profession today. "Lapsus Linguae," for example, is one of the more disturbing explorations of psychoanalysis written from the point of view of both patient and analyst – yet throughout that text, and especially in your concluding comments, you evince great confidence in the potential value of psychoanalysis, and its value for you personally; you also express cautious hope for the ethical future of psychoanalysis. Let me remind you of the following passage:

> psychoanalysis deserves to be construed beyond idealization and demonization, a task to which a judicious skepticism (Harris, 1996) is well suited. Let us acknowledge our collective lapse: psychoanalysis did not protect me, and it has not protected others, from an all too common betrayal, and this failure is very sad. In grieving, of course, I am also claiming psychoanalysis can do better.
>
> (Dimen, 2011, p. 75)

Would you mind elaborating on these thoughts?

Muriel Dimen

It's so interesting to think about idealization. Why does one idealize one's work? Certainly as an anthropologist I did. Is it because in order to endure the work's rigors – whether negotiating hairpin turns with 4000′ drops up to an alpine village at 5000′ where one knows not what will happen, or entering into the work of clinical psychoanalysis that keeps one's mind going at several different levels at once without any guarantee as to outcome – in order to do these hard jobs, one requires a fantasy of the work's perfection? irreplaceability?

Now that I've had two professions, however, I see that skepticism comes more easily. I knew I worshipped one god and it failed, and then I found another, and it too let me down. Surely this is something we are all thought to go through with our parents, although for various reasons I didn't get to do that on time. And with both Dr. O and my second analyst, I didn't get the benefit of disillusionment and repair. (Do we have such a category? Rupture-and-repair is very two-person, crucial to clinical process and intimate relationships. But what about disillusionment-and-repair? Is this book about that?) In my third treatment, conducted at a much slower pace – once a week for many years – I have been able I think to endure the hard knocks of disillusionment, as well as slide into it, while putting things back together again.

So does skepticism emerge from disillusionment-and-repair? Can we know, from the outset, that the shiny thing we love will leave us dry one day, and yet we will be able to love? For I think of skepticism as dry, whereas idealization and demonization are wet with the passions of love and hate, of eros. I do not include thanatos here because I probably know too little about it. Probably we are doing much to avoid its entry into the conversation of SBV, even though it's right there, is it not?

Are SBVs murderous? Mark Blechner points out instances where they are not. Some patients claim them to have been life-giving. So do some analysts, although we tend to suspect them as being self-serving when they say so, protecting either themselves or colleagues or the discipline and its history.

So how do we integrate skepticism into the work? I have in mind a story about a feminist and journalist and her partner/husband, who was one of these supremely self-confident left-wing guys. Their precocious teenager came in one evening to ask whether Gramsci and Marx could be reconciled into one theory. Predictably, the partner/husband launched into an *ex tempore* exegesis, while the feminist journalist said, "Well, that depends."

So when we teach psychoanalysis, can we teach a set of ideas and practices – our praxis – and all along say, "Well, that depends." Might that build in a skepticism? Can we, for example, entertain the idea that successful termination is only more or less complete, is often troubled, incomplete, open for critique?

Does that remove the idealizing glow without substituting the demonizing flame?

Charles Levin

Thank you, I want to linger for a moment on your observations about "disillusionment-and-repair." I love your idea that as analysts we need somehow to integrate skepticism into our work, and that this is far from easy to accomplish. I get the impression that for you disillusionment-and-repair involved a lot of loss and a lot of mourning, without enough environmental support; and that you would like to see this inherently difficult process become less lonely, confusing, and alienating for future generations of young analysts. You mention the possibility of teaching analytic practice in a spirit of moderate reservation that is not overly discouraging for newcomers – the "well, it depends," rather than the supremely self-confident exegesis. I understand you to be saying that there may be a collective psychoanalytic analogy, yet to be realized, of parental renunciation in favor of the child's discovery of desire. What else do you think needs to happen at the level of the analytic group: the discipline, the institution, the community?

Muriel Dimen

This question takes matters in an unexpected direction, and welcomely so. I must say I am rarely comfortable making an analogy from the individual to the group. My reluctance issues from a deeply learned anthropological stance that the individual and the group are two different levels of organization with different principles, dynamics, etc. Can a group have a transference or, for that matter, a countertransference? Are emotions properly ascribed to committees or Houses of Parliament or villages or hospitals? Do such entities dream?

But I will take your question in the spirit in which it is meant: if we think of individual parents and children, then we can think of the individual analysts and candidates who are part of our institutions as borrowing on behaviors, acts, ways of being, and relationships found among parents and children and other individuals.

Now in "Lapsus linguae," I do propose that the parent's renunciation of (incestuous) desire for a child, itself painful to a child as

well as a parent, is crucial to the establishment of desire and difference in the child. My argument is about the centrality of unrequited
love to development. Could it have a similar importance to
training?

Unrequited love – the parent's renunciation and the child's frus-
tration – constitutes the condition on which many losses depend,
hence causes much mourning, anxiety, desire, and creativity. In my
paper, I build on Cooper (2003) and Davies (1998, 2003) to argue
that the analyst's, like the parent's, capacity to refuse the patient's
desires, about which the patient/child is yet unable to think –
indeed, about which the child cannot think sans the parent's renunciation – is the patient's ticket to ride.

Unrequited love grants the room – and I quote myself here –

> to create oneself as if one were autonomous. I am here varying
> Benjamin's (1988) paradox of separation. If independence
> requires separation from the (m)other on whom one depends, so
> claiming one's desire, in all its impossibility and ambiguity, rests
> on having it separately and, in effect, differently from those with
> whom it birthed and still lives – and who understand the pain
> they inflict. If you can reflect on it, unrequited love permits you
> to sense your desire as distinct from, other to, the desire of the
> other who matters to you as much as your own life. But you
> need someone else to help you do it.
>
> (Dimen, 2011, p. 60)

Abjection is one of the main and least tolerable affects of unrequited love and desire. I use this concept in Kristeva's sense of
a corporeal representation of the previously unsymbolized. Sur-
vived – as is usual – abjection creates – quoting myself again – "a
painful, profoundly personal corner for self-knowledge and self-
containment." It creates an opening in which the new can form out
of the inchoate.

> You need to be able to experience your desire, abject and soar-
> ing, with your parent who is feeling this too and knows it and is
> intentionally not acting but is instead bearing the poignant sight
> of your passion as it bursts into flame, you with whom your

parent has identified, whom she or he identifies as her or his own, and whom she or he is allowing to live.

(Dimen, 2011, p. 61)

My prose is a bit purple but it suits the sequelae of rupture. Unrequited love, renunciation, rejection – these are rupturous (my autocorrect tried to change the word to "rapturous") and growth is rough. But one needs them, and that's the reason one needs help.

This brings me to an insight of yours about the struggle I went through. You notice an absence that I hadn't registered: you suggest that for me "disillusionment-and-repair involved a lot of loss and a lot of mourning, without enough environmental support." Perhaps it's true for all of us as we have lived our lacunae: we did not know either that we needed "environmental support" for what we endured, in my case "loss and ... mourning," or that there was, or was allowed, such a thing as provision, let alone a measure such as "enough." That another person has both the sense one is in need, as well as the even more refined sense that such need has its dosage – such a sense would do a lot toward reducing the loneliness, confusion, and alienation one might experience in many situations.

Let me home in on your specific concern: how what we might say here could address training and future analytic generations. I wonder about your observations regarding "the loneliness, confusion, and alienation" of trainees. Do institutes perhaps differ? I believe my own institute generally offers a different experience than most others, and my hunch is confirmed by students of mine as, post-graduation, they engage with the analytic world: they often encounter candidates from other institutes who feel or felt, in their training, constantly reminded of their lowly place. Often their experience was, in effect, if not literally one of being told to keep quiet, an implicit command to subordinate their ideas to those of their teachers and supervisors and, I suppose, analysts.

In my own Institute, candidates have a variety of ways of participating with a fair amount of autonomy, and there are built-in structures that give candidates a say in the running of the institute, with the sense that their voices are heard and respected, that they matter.

I would argue that such in-built balancing of hierarchy constitutes an important part of the foundation for skepticism. If an institute's internal power is grounded in an unquestionable authority structure – in authoritarianism – then skepticism is indeed impossible. Within an authoritarian regime, there's only a paranoid-schizoid mood (yes, I note my use of a concept designed to characterize the individual mind to depict a social entity): if you are not on the side of the institute, or of the powers that be, or of the (current) ruling idea, then you are against it and hence an enemy. Skepticism belongs to intellectual and political structures that allow for more than the two possibilities of "right and wrong." Skepticism is, in contrast, a third place to "yes and no," etc. "It all depends" allows for multiple routes to understanding, multiple and even co-existing perspectives on mind and clinical practices. My Institute has always been home to at least two sorts of psychoanalytic theory, and now there are officially three different theories – and unofficially more – to which one might adhere – or not, because students are not required to pledge allegiance to any one theory, even if faculty are.

Lest I seem to be falling off the edge into idealization, let me make a correction right now. Certainly if one is a candidate at my Institute and wants to have a say in which courses are offered or how faculty are evaluated, it's better to express a theoretical preference and join the group of faculty who identify with it. Without that declaration, one has no structural means to make one's voice heard.

By the same token, for all the democracy and transparency in principle available, there is not only the given, necessary divide in power and authority between faculty and candidates. There is also the sort of informal power structure or hierarchy that graces every institution, and is made of historical relationships and powered by instrumental interests and needs. Even though my institute likes to pride itself on its openness, there are always in-groups and out-groups, there is always excess power to be jockeyed for, and exclusions and inclusions mean that power is inevitably unequally distributed. So while on the face of it skepticism about any particular psychoanalytic set of ideas and clinical practices has a firm grounding in an overtly democratic structure and multiplicity of theoretical perspectives, in lived life identifications with particular ways of thinking and doing create situations in which skepticism, let alone disagreement, can come to seem disloyal.

All this is true of any institution. As analysts, however, we have a particular feature to contend with: those vertical or hierarchical relationships that emerge by virtue of the psychoanalyses candidates undertake as part of their training. Although our candidates are not required to choose as analysts faculty from within our program – they may select anyone who is 5 years or more past graduation from any analytic institute ours recognizes as worthy of the name – and hence the power dynamics issuing from that most personal of relationships, the analytic one, do not necessarily circulate in our institute. Nevertheless many candidates do choose analysts from within the institute, and the complicated loyalties, needs, and fears created by this complex set of forces intensify the obstacles to the emergence of a routine skepticism toward psychoanalysis.

Finally, it is especially when sexual boundary violations come our way that skepticism evaporates. Our institute is no exception to the rule that every institute has been beset by the primal crime. It is noteworthy, however, that when this unfortunate state of affairs eventuated – a state of emergency, one might put it – the inherent offsets to rigid hierarchy that I have described stopped working. It's as though ranks closed, faculty against students against university administration (we are not freestanding, but part of a university) against perpetrators against victims against bystanders against community. During these crises, loneliness, confusion, and alienation reigned, perhaps especially among younger members of the community, and any hierarchy-bridging structures seemed to vanish. Nor was there any room for "it all depends."

But is there ever any such space when it comes to SBVs?

Charles Levin

Let me answer your question with your question! Is there ever a space for reflection and dialogue when it comes to the primal crime? A space for what you describe as disillusionment and repair, for measured deidealization of psychoanalysis? Can you imagine such a space for us? Or are we doomed to cope with these problems as lonely and abject "individuals"?

Muriel Dimen

I have been thinking for a while about this question, and I think I must respond starting at the end. I'm not so sure our coping position is as lonesome, solo, cast aside monads. Our position as individuals who feel the responsibility to fix the problem by ourselves is, in fact, socially constructed. In this unhappy state of mind and being, there is a curious happiness because each of us is indeed part of a group. Each of us is one among many taking on the responsibility assigned us, to figure out something on our own that cannot be figured out alone.

So we inhabit a contradiction which unknowingly we deem it our job to find our way out of. It's kind of like the deadly maze in "The Shining!" We are in a mad sort of system, but a system it is.

There being no socially structured, given way out of it, one way we try to escape is via the informal institution, or practice, known as gossip. Absent any formal structure that can help us cope, we make an effort by talking on the side, indirectly. Following our own informal friendship and collegial networks, we peruse and parse what we know or imagine about a boundary violation. In these recognized but not sanctioned interstices are brief spaces that permit reflection. Such reflection, in singular and general, remains the property of those who arrive at them. It issues from the total context in which the individual as person and category remains privileged, and in effect is a product of that context. But there are no formal channels for holding such reflection(s) in general, in the collective, in shared knowledge, in a public archive.

As it turns out, though, some of the formal structures and processes we do in fact have are now providing spaces toward dialogue, if not always reflection. I am thinking of the panels held, and to be held, and that were planned but did not make it out of the blueprint phase, on the topic at various conferences and institutes across the spectrum of psychoanalytic affiliations. I am thinking of colloquia that have already been offered at institutes, and are in the offing. I am thinking of journals that include papers on this topic, or feature special issues on it. I am thinking of this book.

These are all shared, collective efforts, even if the routes to them may not be described as collective at all. If we have our eye on that particular ball, though, it's possible we may yet stumble on ways to have conversations working toward disillusionment and repair, as I consider you and me to be doing. In the immediate context of sexual boundary violations, reflection and reflective dialogue are nigh-impossible: affect runs too high. On the other hand, if conversations like this take place, are put into the archive, and are available for those who like to think, like this one, then perhaps the space for disillusionment and repair can come more quickly to hand.

Charles Levin

Psychoanalysis was entering a complex new phase in its organizational history when I got involved in the late 1980s. For example, at that time, my society and institute had no official code of ethics. In a sort of public relations panic, and after a bitter fight, we adopted one.

When I heard you present one of the early drafts of "Lapsus Linguae" at a plenary session of the Division 39 meetings in Philadelphia, 2006, I was inspired to think that psychoanalysis is again entering a new era. This time, however, the underlying concern is not so much accountability to the public as accountability to ourselves. Not that the first problem is solved.

There are other ways you have contributed to and changed the ongoing conversation. The metaphor/concept of the "primal crime" strikes me as a linking figure that helps us to mediate between the different levels and domains that concern us – inviting us, for example, to think the individual in the psychoanalytic group and the psychoanalytic group in the individual; and not least, reminding us that there is a whole world "outside" of psychoanalysis, which we cannot simply assimilate or shut out. Your work also suggests another, deeper level to the question of our doctrinal disputes. In the context of the issues you have raised, for example, it seems to me that the term "countertransference" is exposed as the weasel word that it surely is. Beyond the effectiveness of any given technique or theory, which may be considerable, our helpfulness depends upon our growing capacity to "work through" our own troubled subjectivity (in both senses of working through, first as our primary medium and method and secondly as mourning, or "disillusion and repair").

I am posing no particular question here – just floating the magic carpet for you to ride.

Muriel Dimen

Your question sets up the opportunity to think about the relation between psychoanalysis and its context in the same breath as one thinks about the clinical relationship. I will start with a quote from your question: "there is a whole world 'outside' of psychoanalysis, which we cannot simply assimilate or shut out." In an odd way, the perspective in which this statement makes sense is the analytic session, the perspective of analyst and patient sitting together in the quiet of the consulting room, with everything beyond the shut door constituting what you properly put in scare quotes, the "outside." And for that moment this is an apt characterization. We, analyst and patient, are inside, surrounded by something else, which neither requires definition nor, for this slice of time, does it exist.

That's only one time-limited and task-limited perspective, however, which is what your scare quotes signify. The quotation marks tell us that "outside" is a figure of speech as well, and hence has many referents, can signify other things. Or, to put it differently and to keep things perspectival, it can be viewed from other vantage points too. If we think seriously and for any length of time about psychoanalysis as existing apart from this other world, the idea quickly becomes ridiculous. If we view psychoanalysis as a body of knowledge and data, a method of research, and a mode of treatment or cure – as Freud did – then we have to consider it as an entity and set of processes with a history, a social place, and practitioners. Think of Makari's excellent *Revolution in Mind* (2008), which shows not only how psychoanalytic thought evolved within medicine and psychology but within Freud's life, and how psychoanalysis fared in and affected its medium.

Often psychoanalytic writers attempt to acknowledge this "outside" world by referring to the "social surround." That locution irritates me no end. As if psychoanalysis were a thing encircled by, but not of, the "social." I guess what annoys me about that phrase is that it constitutes an attempt at what you so wisely call "assimilation." It's kind of a speech act that acts as though we psychoanalysts really do know about the significance and force of the cultural and, having named it, need pay it no further attention. The very naming, the putative acknowledgement, is in effect an erasure.

The world psychoanalysis inhabits is not a surround. It's a medium. It is the stuff of which any practice – psychoanalysis, medicine, art – is made. You could say it's shot through with this "outside" world, laced with culture. But that's to take the material that's riddled with culture as though it were not itself cultural *ab initio.*

So how do we psychoanalysts, indeed, how does psychoanalysis, find a way to talk about, think through, and make use of that of which it created? In the social sciences, it's commonly accepted that one cannot step outside the medium one inhabits: our view of what we are and do emerges from what we do and are. There is no Archimedean point from which to understand and depict our medium, which means we have to start from the middle of where we are.

Your question suggests a way of doing this. I quote: "In the context of the issues you have raised, for example, it seems to me that the term 'countertransference' is exposed as the weasel word that it surely is." Now I'm not sure what you intend by "weasel," and perhaps in your reply you will expand. But you point to the perspective implicit in the term: the very notion of "counter" transference issues from the perspective of that aspect of psychoanalysis called by some a "one-person" psychology, which is itself a cultural product based on a view of human existence as though it emerges from and proceeds through persons living as monads, not as members of social groups and institutions. The analyst's set of feelings and thoughts and stances toward the patient "counter" what the patient brings: the patient initiates it all.

I need not rehearse here the critique at the foundation of relational psychoanalysis. My point is that at various locations on the map of psychoanalysis it is currently being recognized that "counter" transference suggests a response to a state of mind that originates within another person: you react to me as though I'm your father and, should I have paternal feelings toward you, they issue from you, not from me nor, more important for our discussion, the space between us.

The notion of "counter" refuses admission to the conceptual arma-
mentarium the idea of what we now call the intersubjective. My unconscious, preconscious, and conscious feelings, thoughts, and fantasies
about you, like yours about me, are already in being in the space – psychic, cultural, symbolic – holding us, preceding us, re-created and
altered by us as we live in it. The intersubjective renders the question
of who started it – your/my transference or my/your "counter" transference – useless for us as both thinkers and clinicians. None of us has
the power to start or stop it. All we can do is be in its midst, inscribed
by and reinscribing it in our own way.

What is useful is to think about how each party to the dyad
behind the closed door brings into that quiet the "troubled subjectivities," as you call them, that have their origin simultaneously in
personal history and in mutually meaningful contexts that say there
exist such things as "trouble," that troubled and untroubled minds
can be found, and suggest it is both possible and good to search for
untroubled minds and the source of trouble, and aspire toward
a state of untroubledness. Here we enter Harry Stack Sullivan's territory: we are all more human than otherwise and, of the two in the
consulting room, one, relatively well, is trying to help the other,
who is relatively ill.

Yet we also exceed Sullivan. Your formulation of the knots we are
trying to disentangle proposes that notions of well-being and of ill-
health are culturally situated. Therefore we are required to inquire:
of what might an untroubled subjectivity consist? Given that intersubjective space contains more than one mind, is it possible that the
multiplicity of subjectivities guarantees trouble? Otherness, that
elemental constituent of intersubjectivity, means difficulty for each
of us: not only the Other outside us but the Other within makes for
troubled subjectivities. If I enter treatment with the idea of
a sexualized father-daughter relation in which the sexuality is
stoutly denied, I am in trouble already. I bring in an entirely familiar cultural configuration that makes for trouble all the time unless
it is recognized and named in such a way as not to be assimilated
and erased but maintained as a necessary object of ongoing investigation. I am in trouble not only in relation to Dr. O but in relation
to my internal Other who is entangled in this filial sexualization,
happily and miserably. Not to mention my relation to the Other in

Dr. O, who treated his Otherness as though it had never distorted the treatment.

Therefore it is incumbent on us, as we notice, create, enact, and unpack the phenomena we call transference and "counter" transference to understand how they embody the "outside." In other words, the mutual attention analyst and patient pay to their entanglement with each other, an attention meant to clarify, cure, and recontextualize their respective troubles, is how the "outside" is already "inside". The exploration of the analyst's troubled subjectivity along with that of the patient's takes place because the dyad is not surrounded by culture, it is in and of it already, it embodies and recreates and puts new spins on it all the time. The call-and-response animating the dyad is a figure of social being each party has already partaken of before the first consultation is even set up. The analytic ethic according to which the analyst must self-analyze as part of analyzing the patient is given by their shared origins in the fact of human culture, the fact that we are always already in relation to one another and to the Others within and without, that such necessarily troubled relations are as vital to human going-on-being as food, water, shelter, and words.

References

Benjamin, J. (1988). *The bonds of love.* New York: Pantheon.

Cooper, S.H. (2003). You say Oedipal, I say postOedipal. *Psychoanalytic Dialogues* 13: 41–63.

Davies, J.M. (1998). Between the disclosure and the foreclosure of erotic transference-countertransference: Can psychoanalysis find a place for adult sexuality? *Psychoanalytic Dialogues* 8: 747–766.

Davies, J.M. (2003). Falling in love with love. *Psychoanalytic Dialogues* 13: 1–27.

Dimen, M. (2011). Lapsus linguae, or a slip of the tongue? A sexual violation in an analytic treatmetn and its personal and theoretical aftermath. *Contemporary Psychoanalysis* 47(1): 35–79.

Harris, A. (1996). The anxiety in ambiguity: Reply to Brenneis, Crews, and Stern. *Psychoanalytic Dialogues* 6(2): 267–279.

Makari, G. (2008). *Revolution in mind: The creation of psychoanalysis.* New York: Harper.

Index

Morrison, S. 89
Moses 8, 202–208
mother-child relationships 53, 68, 206
mourning 111, 224, 226, 230
murder 7
mutual analysis 155
mutual co-construction of belief 160
mutual feelings 116

narcissism: and the avoidance of shame
82; collective 7, 207, 209; father-son
projective identification 201; folk
theories 31; and incest 198;
institutions of psychoanalysis 23;
of the law 191–194; malignant
narcissistic leader figure 212; in the
Moses story 203, 204, 205; narcissistic
boundary violation 14–15; narcissistic
fantasy 112; narcissistic predators 37;
narcissistic protections 213–214; and
power 14–15; and sovereignty 205,
207; submissive narcissism 212
nation-building 5–6
negative capability 140–141
negative hallucinations 19
neoliberalism 83
neurosis 46, 50, 53, 140, 212
Nietzsche, F. 134–135, 139
non-admission of guilt 94
nonverbal communication 156, 157
not-me 120
nuclear complex 192
nurturing (versus appropriating) desire 21

object hunger 71
object relations 103, 111, 157, 164
objectivity 199
Oedipal dynamics: in the analytic
relationship 53; collective 208;
institutions of psychoanalysis 67;
nuclear complex 192; separation from
incest taboo 22, 179; and the sexual in
sexual boundary violations 102–103,
112, 177, 178–179, 180, 182
Ogden, T. 145, 156
Oliver, Kelly 82, 94
ombudsman 57
omnipotence 70–72, 111, 135,
196–197, 203
one-person psychology 5, 232
one-time offender theories 31
ostracization from the group 10, 49, 53,
74, 94

other spaces 152
otherness 74, 82, 90, 93, 120, 156–158,
161–163, 209, 233

painful growth 15
panopticon 159, 163
paranoid-schizoid position 111, 227
Parat, C.J. 140
parent-child relationships 178–180, 201,
224, 233; see also fathers; mother-child
relationships
Parsons, M. 138, 140, 142
patients, analysts as 176, 181, 199; see
also personal analysis
patient-victims 9
patriarchy 4, 7, 8, 88, 183, 192, 194, 197,
200–201, 202, 203, 205
Pellegrini, Ann 22, 175–189
Peltz, R. 152, 154
perpetrator perspectives 9, 45–60
personal analysis 13, 35, 119, 199
personal information, analyst disclosing
46, 47
perverse carefulness 20
perversity 65–66, 157–162, 163, 196, 209
phantasmatic scenes 161, 163
phantasy 208
Phillips, Adam 32, 110, 111, 175,
176, 180
Pinsky, E. 61, 110, 114
pith and kith 1
Plato 2, 7, 23, 197–200, 205, 207
play 136
police 81, 87–88
policing of analytic bodies 37, 77
political history of psychoanalysis 195
pollution 34–36, 37, 39
pollution fears 30
polymorphous nature of adult
sexuality 196
post-analytic meetings, inappropriate
46, 47
post-colonial theory 82
post-structuralism 21
power: in the analytic relationship 176;
asymmetry 147, 155, 159, 201; and
authority 91, 137, 195, 199, 205, 207,
227; binaries of 152; and the body 156;
and consent 83; disciplinary 177–178;
and fantasy 163; father figures 203;
and the field of psychoanalysis 151;
and hatred 40; and identification 194;
institutions of psychoanalysis 227; and